YOUR SMILE IS A WORK OF ART

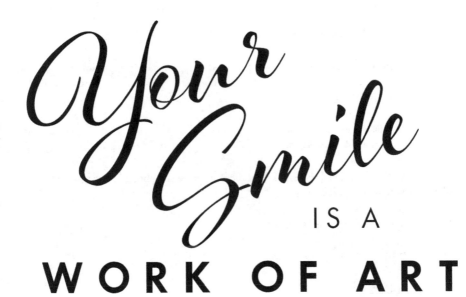

Your Smile IS A WORK OF ART

CHANGING THE WAY YOU THINK ABOUT DENTISTRY

GREGORY J. WYCH, DDS

Advantage®

Published by Advantage, Charleston, South Carolina.
Member of Advantage Media Group.

ADVANTAGE is a registered trademark, and the Advantage colophon is a trademark of Advantage Media Group, Inc.

Printed in the United States of America.

10 9 8 7 6 5 4 3 2 1

ISBN: 978-1-64225-048-0
LCCN: 2018950242

Cover design by Melanie Cloth.
Layout design by Megan Elger.

This publication is designed to provide accurate and authoritative information in regard to the subject matter covered. It is sold with the understanding that the publisher is not engaged in rendering legal, accounting, or other professional services. If legal advice or other expert assistance is required, the services of a competent professional person should be sought.

Advantage Media Group is proud to be a part of the Tree Neutral® program. Tree Neutral offsets the number of trees consumed in the production and printing of this book by taking proactive steps such as planting trees in direct proportion to the number of trees used to print books. To learn more about Tree Neutral, please visit **www.treeneutral.com**.

Advantage Media Group is a publisher of business, self-improvement, and professional development books and online learning. We help entrepreneurs, business leaders, and professionals share their Stories, Passion, and Knowledge to help others Learn & Grow. Do you have a manuscript or book idea that you would like us to consider for publishing? Please visit **advantagefamily.com** or call **1.866.775.1696**.

TABLE OF CONTENTS

INTRODUCTION

I grew up in Cleveland, Ohio, and since I was young, dentistry had always been on my mind. I went to undergrad at Xavier University in Cincinnati, where I experienced my biggest dental woe—but also one that changed how I thought about dentistry. During an intense game of racquetball, my friend accidentally smacked me in the face with his racquet, breaking a lot of my front teeth.

I borrowed a buddy's car and drove up to Cleveland to see my family dentist. He opted for a lot of bonding, using tooth-colored composite resins to repair my front teeth. At the time, it seemed like all was well—until I realized that, over the years, the bonding wasn't very strong, and I constantly broke them.

I struggled with these bondings for up to eight years. During that time, I attended and graduated from dental school at Case Western Reserve University in Cleveland, and immediately joined the Navy afterward. I was stationed down in Beaufort at Parris Island Marine Corps Recruit Depot, and also at the Marine Corps Air Station—there's a large military presence in South Carolina, especially with retired veterans, so I always find it a treat when I'm able to interact to servicemen and women.

After I finished my service, I worked as an associate for a dentist in Columbia, South Carolina, where I sought to remain after my time in the Navy—keep in mind I still had bondings on my front teeth that broke quite often. This dentist was adamant about placing veneers on my front teeth. Now, this guy was a very good general dentist, and an expert on root canals, and crowns, and fillings— he could do all of that very well. But despite his skillset, cosmetic dentistry was still in its infancy at the time, which led to unfavorable results. The veneers were a mess. I'd break them all the time and try to fix them myself in the mirror—none of it was working for me. I had to deal with that for quite a while.

A few years later, still donning the dentist's veneers, I established my own practice in Irmo, and that practice has been in the same location since 1996.

And still, through dental school, the Navy, working in a dentist's office as an associate, and finally building my own practice, my front teeth were still a thorn in my side. I was a dentist, overseeing patients and ushering them into a healthier lifestyle via dental hygiene—and I couldn't even get my own teeth to look the way I wanted!

So around the time I opened the Irmo location in 1996, I was doing a lot of continuing education in cosmetic dentistry and heard about a very well-known dentist named Bill Dickerson, who practiced out in Las Vegas. I took the trip and paid full fee for him to restore my veneers. And just like that, the veneers lasted for over twenty years.

I always tell people I paid full fee for these veneers because, at the time, I was going through a lot of hardships in my life. I was getting divorced, losing a lot of stuff, and in general, it shouldn't have been a time where a person would typically invest in themselves. But I've always been into self-improvement and finding ways to better myself. So, remembering the ideas of Jim Rohn, who always used to push the notion of investing in yourself, I decided to get these veneers done.

Recently, I chose to get my veneers redone for a second time. The ones Bill Dickerson had done for me had lasted for over twenty years, so I was looking for another long-lasting solution for my front teeth. I teach at dental seminars several times a year in Scottsdale, Arizona at a dental institute called the Spear Institute, and during one visit, I made the decision to ask Gary DeWood, one of the founding members of Spear, to redo my veneers. Again, I paid full fee because I was confident in his ability and trusted that I would be getting the best veneers possible, and if that's anything to go by, I'll probably have these veneers on for the rest of my life!

I share my own dental journey with others because I want to emphasize the value of self-improvement. I believe that is core to dentistry as a whole. Over everything else, people want to invest in themselves and improve their smile, whether that is through cosmetic dentistry or by learning proper dental hygiene and maintenance.

As a society, we tend to judge people very quickly, within the first few seconds—and research by Kelton Global on behalf of the American Academy of Cosmetic Dentistry shows 48 percent of adults think a smile is the most memorable feature on first impressions with people. To add to this, 37 percent of the participants in the study found flawed smiles to be less attractive than those with perfect smiles.[1] This includes anyone from an athlete who might've

---

1   "Best Face Forward: Making GREAT First Impressions in a Digital Age," Surveys & Research, American Academy of Cosmetic Dentistry, date accessed May 9, 2018, https://www.aacd.com/proxy/files/Publications%20and%20Resources/AACD_First_Impressions.pdf

suffered an unfortunate accident (like I had) to a parent who put their children's needs before their own, and wants to finally get the dental work they've always wanted. So, for many adults who enter my practice, they are striving for self-improvement in their lives—and the first step is having a dentist they can really trust.

HOW CAN YOU TELL IF A DENTIST IS QUALIFIED?

For the amount of people who seek self-improvement through their smiles, they tend to do themselves a disservice by not researching their dentists before going to their practice. Throughout my thirty-three years of dental experience, I've seen firsthand how patients are too eager to choose dentists that may not have the correct experience to provide the results they want to achieve.

I tell students the same story a lot. It revolves around this older woman who called into the office, requesting to see my associate dentist on a day that I wasn't in the office. When she got to the office and met with the office assistant, she pulled out a newspaper from her purse and showed us an ad my practice had run a few months ago, which was actually the ad spot I had bought that welcomed my associate to my practice. The woman said, "I've had this ad for nine months, and I really like the way she looks in this picture. I figured since she was fresh out of dental school, she knew all the newest techniques—I want her to be my dentist!"

The woman later came back for a cleaning with the hygienist, and the associate dentist came in to place an upper partial denture—she ended up messing it up completely. I had to come into work and fix it for the patient, teaching my associate the entire time about the treatment and walking her through how to do it properly. Eventually, word did get out that I was the one who completed the treatment, not my associate, and the patient confessed she only wanted to see me from that moment forward. I listen to all my patients, and make sure that I am the one in charge of fulfilling all of their needs.

That story always stuck with me because I think people are too quick to make judgements on important life decisions, dentistry being no exception. When you're trusting your teeth and bite to a dentist, you're going to want to make sure they are the most experienced and confident choice around you.

A great dentist will be someone that participates in continuing education—as technology constantly evolves—along with keeping up with the newest techniques and treatment methods. If a dentist is not up-to-date on the latest advancements in the field, then that is a dentist you do not want working on your treatment. In addition, a great dentist is also a teacher, and most will teach at a nearby dental school or lecture at seminars. Personally, I continue to stay on top of continuing education and provide the most up-to-date services at my practice, and as I mentioned earlier, I am part of the visiting faculty at the Spear Institute in Arizona.

Another great thing to ask for when considering a dentist is their case history, experience, and before and after photos. Most dentists should have a plethora of before and after pictures to show you, especially if it relates to your case. This will allow you to see how the results turned out, and it will be an opportunity for the dentist to further explain the steps to achieve that desired result.

Lastly, a great dentist will focus on specific things in his or her practice. Instead of trying to do it all—a dentist that tries to be a jack-of-all-trades but a master of none—a great dentist knows his strengths and will seek to make that the core of the office. Of course, a general dentist should be able to perform treatments like root canals and crowns—the basics—but others, for a lack of a better term, specialize in certain areas. For example, my practice focuses heavily on cosmetic and sedation dentistry—that's something we hang our hats on.

I always tell my patients if you're used to being Scotch-taped and patched, a lot of guys can do that. But if you're looking for something that is going to last, then maybe you need to just be more specific in your research.

THE ART OF DENTISTRY

My dental practice, The Art of Dentistry, has been in the same location in Irmo since 1996, just twelve miles outside of Columbia, South Carolina. When I started this practice, I wanted to differentiate myself from other dental offices—especially the corporate practices that litter many cities in America. Those practices are just focused on their patient intake and the amount of money they're able to make off of drilling and filling teeth day-to-day.

When you walk into my practice, you'll first notice the amount of expensive art hanging on the walls—I've spent a small fortune just for this art alone. I want patients and prospective patients to feel like they're in somewhere luxurious, because there's no greater luxury than their health. After speaking to the office assistant—who will make you feel right at home by offering tea, coffee or a cool drink (even a healthy snack)—you can relax in the Tempur-Pedic cushioned chairs. Even when it's time to go to the examination room, you'll be able to relax while I am working on your teeth.

However, I understand that many people are fearful to go to the dentist and can't relax despite our best efforts. This fear can range from slight stress and uncomfortableness to intense claustrophobia and panic attacks. This dental anxiety is actually very well documented, with estimations of up to 15 percent of Americans having some sort of dental anxiety, which leads them to avoid the dentist because of it.[2] That's up to 48 million people that are suffering from fear of the dentist! With most of my patients, this dental anxiety arose from bad experiences with previous dentists.

I try to make the patient as comfortable as possible, and I always call them the night before their appointment to talk about any questions or concerns they have regarding the morning's visit, and to formally welcome them into the practice. However, even if it's just for a cleaning, some patients are too claustrophobic or too scared to sit in the chair and get their work done. To combat this dental anxiety, my practice offers sedation dentistry. I don't think there's anybody, at least in the counties around me, that even have permits for sedation dentistry, which makes us a unique practice in the area. Specifically, we market a lot for moderate oral sedation, which really helps patients relax and get their case done without the typical fears associated with dentistry. Eventually, as the patient grows more and more comfortable with the office and my work, they sometimes choose to push through without sedation, and it's always great to see them make progress with their fears. I'll speak a little bit more about the different types of sedation dentistry in chapter ten.

Once the patient is relaxed, whether it is through the spa-like atmosphere or necessary oral sedation, then we'll be able to get their treatment started. I look for solutions in many modes of treatment, whether that be fixing a patient's bite with Invisalign or creating a perfect smile through the use of dental implants. My practice has all the latest technology, and everything is up-to-date, so there's no need to be worried about "newer" treatment techniques—we already have

---

2   "What is Dental Anxiety and Phobia?" Colgate, date accessed May 9, 2018, https://www.colgate.com/en-us/oral-health/basics/dental-visits/what-is-dental-anxiety-and-phobia

it! One of my favorite modes of treatment comes in the form of Fast Braces, an alternative to traditional braces.

I was the first dentist provider of Fast Braces in South Carolina, and have reached the level of Senior Master Affiliate with the appliance—the only one in South Carolina and Georgia—so, suffice it to say, I have a lot of experience with it and recommend them to many patients, especially those who urgently need the work braces can provide, but in a shorter time frame. This happens frequently with men and women who are getting married soon and can't afford to be in braces for two years. Fast Braces can get the work done in half the time, and sometimes even less than that.

Aside from a variety of services we provide, one of the things my patients love the most is our dedication to dental photography. We always take high-resolution before-and-after pictures of our patients so we can share them with other prospective patients. We also make sure to document pictures of the treatment process so we can use those to help educate our patients on what exactly they will be going through—the selected mode of treatment, the steps they need to take along with us to secure that treatment, and the steps they need to take to make sure that the treatment lasts a lifetime. We've done these types of consultations for everything from standard braces to oral surgeries. It doesn't matter if it's a simple problem or a complex problem—the best way for the patient to understand their options is to educate them every step of the way.

And most patients I see that come in have complex problems over simple ones. A lot of people don't realize how important dental hygiene is until the problem is already starting to spiral out of control. Folks will come in with a multitude of cavities or they'll have temporomandibular joint dysfunction (TMD)—problems with the jaw joints—or sometimes will be missing teeth entirely. They'll wait for all of these red flags before scheduling an appointment with me. So when I'm treating patients, I not only go over their specific case, but I make sure they're aware of how incredibly important oral health is in general, especially in how it affects your overall health and body—in fact, tooth loss is associated with a shorter life span.[3] There's also a lot of correlation between people who have diabetes or cardiology issues and people who have poor oral hygiene.

I try to make this all clear to my patients, not to scare them, but because I genuinely care for their health and want them to succeed with a great smile. I'll send handwritten notes and mail them off to patients constantly wishing them well and checking in on them, especially if they've had lingering problems for a while. They all have my personal e-mail and cell phone number, so even if they have questions on a weekend that can't wait, they can reach me. Again, I genuinely care about my patients—and not just the ones that walk into my office.

We participate in giving back to the local community, and are partners with a program called Give Back a Smile through the American Academy of Cosmetic Dentistry (AACD). Give Back a Smile is a charitable foundation that was created to restore the smiles of men and women that are victims of domestic and sexual violence and abuse from a former intimate partner, spouse or family member.

I've done many of these cases throughout the years, more than any other dentist in the area, and I believe it's one of the more important aspects of dentistry. There's already a great feeling when I'm able to see the impact my work has on patients, and the feeling becomes indescribable when helping these men and women get a

---

3   Paula K. Friedman and Ira B. Lamster, "Tooth loss as a predictor of shortened longevity: exploring the hypothesis," *Periodontology 2000* 72, no. 1 (October 2016): 142–152, https://doi.org/10.1111/prd.12128

smile they've always wanted. It boosts their self-confidence and gives them opportunities they wouldn't have had otherwise.

This all comes full-circle back to how my practice operates. We're all about the Disney style and Ritz-Carlton level of customer service. From the moment you walk through our doors to the second you leave the practice, we want to be sure you are comfortable, and have a reason to smile.

IT'S NOT TOO LATE TO TAKE CHARGE OF YOUR ORAL HEALTH

Yes, sometimes it can be a chore to keep up with your dental hygiene. I even know a lot of dentists who don't manage to brush twice a day, or floss daily. The key is constantly drilling the good habits of brushing twice a day and flossing daily so you maintain the healthiness of your teeth and gums. And of course, the most important thing you can do is to visit the dentist twice a year and follow their instructions closely, especially if you have any issues.

Don't fall for do-it-yourself fixes or strange, natural remedies you see online. Honestly—I've had some patients come into my practice with horrible problems, and when I ask when's the last time they saw a dentist, they couldn't tell me. Instead, they sought to improve their own oral hygiene in different ways, using methods that are unproven and just can't replace brushing and flossing. A popular thing going around right now is "oil pulling," where a person swishes oil in their mouth for fifteen to twenty minutes, which is apparently supposed to be good for the gums and teeth. There's nothing really concrete to back this up, and even if there were—*why not just brush and floss?* This is akin to the old belief that putting aspirin next to a toothache would help ease the pain, when in reality, all it resulted in were burns from the acidity of the aspirin! Now, is oil pulling going to harm you? No, probably not. But if you depend on it as a substitute for proper oral hygiene of brushing and flossing, then you're going to end up with bigger problems than you started with.

All of this is to say—go to the dentist. Even if you feel your teeth are perfect—you haven't had a cavity ever and your teeth are straight and white—a skilled dentist will be able to determine if something is wrong that you may not have even noticed was there. Problems don't just get better on their own, they get way worse, and it will end up costing you more in the long run. Get your teeth looked at by a professional dentist, sooner rather than later.

It's never too late to take your health into your own hands. Especially when you're an adult, who most of my patients tend to be, and your children have grown up and are taking care of themselves— you still have the opportunity to improve your quality of life. The best investment you can make is in yourself, no matter if you're just beginning your professional career, or on the brink of retirement.

Over the past thirty-three years, I have helped well over five thousand patients with implant, sedation and cosmetic dentistry. I am passionate about helping my patients love their teeth, and take their oral health seriously so their overall health and quality of life never suffers. I want the best for you, and I hope that by reading this book, you'll want the best for yourself, too!

CHAPTER 1

Why Read This Boring Little Book?

Let's be honest, there are a lot more exciting things you could spend your time reading. You know that, I know that, and anyone who sees what you are reading knows that, too. It's not every day that people recommend a book about choosing a dentist. They don't hit the bestseller lists, and nobody is lined up to turn it into a movie. Having said all of that, there are still some really good reasons to read this boring little book.

When it comes to you and your family, you want what is best for them. But what you may not realize is that without nice teeth and a great smile, you all may not go as far in life. The truth of the matter is that kids who have teeth problems tend to fall behind, be bullied, lack confidence, and get lower grades. What child wants to stand in front of the classroom to speak when they have teeth that people laugh at? Adults who have teeth problems can have trouble concentrating at work, miss time at the job, and suffer needlessly every day.

Life is tough, and with tooth pain, or worse—a less than awesome smile—people judge you without really knowing you. Did you know that people who don't know you will form their opinion about you in less than the first second when you walk into a room?[4] Helping your family get their best start in life includes making sure they have excellent dental care.

Social shaming and bullying is more common, degrading, and persistent than when we were kids. Teen suicide is at record levels and on the rise, and such events share this one thing in common: shocked and bewildered parents who could not conceive of their kid ending his own life. Sure, they noticed he was a little depressed. They knew some kids were making fun of him. Yes, she started spending more time home, alone, not coming out of her room, but she is a teenager. What once was a few days or weeks of misery contained with a few bullies in the cafeteria is now endless, expansive, broadcast online, and far nastier than most would dare commit in person. And if you don't think being a buck-toothed girl or boy with crooked teeth is enough to set off a massive assault of this sort, you are frankly not in touch at all with what these kids are doing to each other online.

Going to junior high with crooked teeth and a humiliating smile is one thing. Hey, plenty of kids are going to school without shoes. So, why are teeth such a big deal? Beyond just high school, your children will go on college admission interviews, head off to college, go on job interviews—trying to fit into these new and anxiety rich environments at a faraway place while dealing with a bad smile,

---

4   Janine Willis and Alexander Todorov, "First impressions: making up your mind after a 100-ms exposure to a face," *Psychol Sci* 17, no.7 (July 2006): 592–8, https://doi.org/10.1111/j.1467-9280.2006.01750.x

unavoidable bad breath, or daytime headaches from nighttime teeth-grinding is a lot more serious.

As an adult, we are looking to improve ourselves and be more successful. Our loved ones depend on us to do this. Yet, with dental pain, or a smile that holds us back, we are destined to struggle to get ahead. So many adults suffer because they are missing the confidence that a great smile can give.

Regardless of our job or profession, we all have to deal with the public and sell ourselves every day. Without that great smile, we start out behind the eight ball. Our dental health even affects our social behavior. I can't tell you how many times a spouse will tell me that they have become social hermits for fear of losing or breaking their teeth, even their teeth falling out in public. Dentures, partials, worn or missing teeth can really paralyze an adult and even their spouse.

Patients have told me they never realized how important it was to wake up with teeth in their mouth, until they were waking up next to someone they loved.

While it may not be the most exciting thing to read, dentistry can have a major impact on your own life and your children's. Everyone wants and needs a nice smile, nobody wants their teeth to be in pain, and choosing the right dentist for you and your family can quite honestly make a world of difference. It only takes one time sitting in the dentist's chair and not feeling comfortable about what is taking place to know how important choosing the right dentist is. It just takes looking in the mirror and not liking the teeth you see to realize that having the right dentist at your side can impact your life in many ways.

As a dentist, I know what it's like to have a broken smile. Like I mentioned in the introduction, I know what it is like to suffer with a broken smile. But I also know what a great, expertly restored smile can do for you. And I treat many phobic patients with sedation dentistry, as I know the stories and the fears that many folks have with the dentist.

But this book is not about me, or what I do, it's about you and the decisions you make and how they can help or harm your life. I've come in contact with thousands of people, and I've seen how important it is to choose the right dentist and to know how to get the best out of your whole dental experience.

How much would you say you trust your dentist? Trust is a huge factor when it comes to your dentist. You need to trust that the person will suggest treatments that you really need, rather than ones that will simply line their pockets. Are you tired of walking out of the dental office with a big bill in your hand, and a huge question in your heart as to whether or not you really needed all that work to begin with? Having a dentist you trust is crucial to getting care that you will feel comfortable with.

Remember when you were a child and your parents took you to either the only dentist in town or they just grabbed one from the phone book? Nobody paid much attention to what dentist they went to, and most people didn't know why it mattered at all anyway. It created a generation of people who feared the dentist, because they often had poor experiences. I'm here to tell you that you don't have to worry so much. You can relax.

Today we realize how important it is to choose the right dentist. Not every dentist makes a good fit for every person, and vice versa.

If you want to have the best possible experience, you have to take the time to learn about what makes a great dentist, how to go about choosing one, and what you can expect from them.

I've written this book to take the guesswork out of the equation. I know it can be confusing to choose a dentist. Do you choose based off location? How about their experience and specialties? What about those offering a coupon to get me in the door? These are all legitimate questions and they are often part of what goes into why people choose the dentist they choose. But are these questions good enough? The short answer is no, there's more that needs to go into it.

Once you finish reading this book, you will have a good sense of what makes for a good dentist, why choosing the right one should matter to you, and where to begin your search.

For many people, the right dentist may come along only once in a lifetime. When they move out of reach of that dentist, or if the dentist retires, the person may feel as though no other dentist can replace them. That's how much you want to love your dentist. You want to feel like there's nobody who could replace that person because they make you feel that they care about you as a patient, they have your best interest at heart, and they are one-of-a-kind in the field.

It's also important to realize that a lot has changed over the years when it comes to dentistry. While you may have memories from your childhood of going to the dentist and it being scary, the technology has come a long way. Sit in the dentist's chair today and you will see all the high-tech equipment used to quickly get pictures of your teeth, fill cavities, and apply fluoride. Even procedures like root canals are so much easier than they were in the past. Just like medicine, everything is better today than it was when we were kids.

A lot has changed in dentistry over the years, making it a much more patient-friendly experience.

There are a lot of things that people worry about when it comes to choosing a dentist. They have their initial fears that there's going to be pain involved—a lot of pain. Then there are the fears about how much work will be needed, if the dentist is qualified to do all that is needed, and how much the bill is going to be. Then there are added fears about being able to schedule appointments around work or school, and other added stressors.

These are quite honestly issues that you don't have to worry about, and my hope is I'll help you to see that. Dentistry is quite painless today because modern technology has addressed that issue. Plus, we can offer a variety of payment options to help you be able to comfortably afford any treatment you may need. Your first priority should be to get the treatment that you need, not spend time worrying about paying for it. That is usually solved without any issues.

I've known numerous patients who started out needing to have a small cavity filled. They put it off, for whatever reason, thinking that by delaying the treatment they were putting off expenses and the work. The problem with this is that the cavity continues to get worse. Then you have a bigger cavity that needs to be filled, and the bigger the cavity, the more you are risking needing a crown, which will add even more to the treatment expense.

Simply taking care of the issue at hand as soon as it's identified can help keep costs down. Going to the dentist twice per year for your check-ups and cleanings can also lower expenses, because you'll maintain your teeth's health. Regular dental cleanings will stave off plaque from teeth and can go a long way toward helping keep your teeth and gums healthy for years.

Some patients just give up hope. They have so many problems—broken, loose or missing teeth—that they just stay away from the dentist because they think it is too late, or they are too far gone to be able to afford the treatment. But did you know, that Dr. Mayo, of the Mayo Clinic said that losing your teeth could actually cost you up to ten years of your life?

The bottom line is that if you want to be able to smile and laugh without trying to cover your mouth up out of embarrassment, that doesn't just happen on its own. You need to have a dentist you can trust who will help guide you, identify where there are issues and help you find the best treatment, and help you feel comfortable.

WHY CHOOSING THE RIGHT DENTIST IS A MUST

1. You and your family want to feel comfortable and confident every time you go to the dentist. You can only have that comfort if you know you have the right dentist for you.

2. Your smile is the first thing that most people notice about you. It's also the cornerstone of your confidence. Loving your smile is essential to feeling confident talking to people, laughing in front of others, and in loving what you see when you look in the mirror.

3. Having the right dentist for you means that you will always be able to get the appointments you need. You won't have to stress about how to fit them into your schedule or try to take off work or school to always get them done.

4. You will know that you have a dentist that keeps up with the changes in the industry, and uses advanced technology in order to bring you the most comfortable experience.

5.   You will know that the dentist you choose has a great reputation and is well respected. The dentist will have a track record of being great with other patients, helping you feel more comfortable about what they can do for you and your family.

6.   You want your kids to grow up feeling good about who they are and how they look, rather than having teeth that have problems that lead them to being bullied. You want to feel confident when you shake hands with someone in the office, and you want your kids to no longer be embarrassed when they get called to the front of the classroom to give a presentation.

We have all known someone who covers their mouth up when they laugh in a crowd. Or maybe they don't want to show their teeth when they smile. Or maybe they suffer needlessly with dental pain. They may even be the child who hides in the back of the room, afraid to go before his peers because he doesn't like his teeth. Whether we realize it or not, how we feel about our teeth plays a major role in how we feel about ourselves as a whole.

I can't emphasize enough that how you feel about your teeth helps to lay the foundation for how you feel about yourself overall. It also helps others to form their opinion about you. While adults may be a bit kinder when it comes to someone who has problems with their teeth or smile, children are not. Let's be honest in saying that they can be absolutely brutal.

If you feel bad or embarrassed about how your teeth look or feel, then there's a good chance you will suffer. You won't want to smile, participate, laugh, or do many of the things we associate with happiness and being successful. Being happy with the teeth and smile you have makes a major difference in your life.

When you have teeth and a smile that you love and are comfortable with, you are more inclined to:

- Be happier with yourself and in life in general. When you love the way your teeth look, you will find yourself more able to smile and be happy.

- Speak up, speak out, and participate more. You will no longer be the adult hiding in the back of the boardroom, or the child who hides in the back of the classroom.

- Have more confidence in everything you do. People who love their teeth and smile will smile more, coming across as friendly. They may find that they speak to more people have more relationships as a result.

Being confident with your teeth makes you more confident in life, which helps you do more, achieve more, and have more fun. It all comes down to finding the right dentist and putting your trust in the person to help you have the best teeth and smile going forward.

If you are like me, and like most other people in the country, you want to be happy. Smiling tends to make people happier, and being happier leads to being more positive. We can all use some more positivity in our lives. Research shows that when we smile more there are many things that take place, including: lowering your stress level and negative thinking patterns, as well as increasing your attention span and productivity.

It may be hard to believe that so much is weighted on a smile, but it really is. Our smile is not only something we notice about ourselves, but it's also one of the first impressions others have of us. And you know how important first impressions can be. A smile has a major impact on such things as getting hired for a job, being more easily remembered, others finding us attractive, and more. Most people conducting interviews know within the first seconds of meeting the person whether or not they are in the running for the position. The smile says it all. Flash a smile that has crooked, dull teeth that are filled with stains and plaque and you can kiss that job goodbye.

When you smile, your brain releases dopamine, serotonin, and endorphins, which are "feel good" neurotransmitters. They help relieve stress and pain and keep you feeling good and happy. These neurotransmitters give us more confidence, and the ability to cope better in life. Smiles are also contagious, with people often unconsciously responding to a smile with a smile. As you can see, the importance of our smile goes beyond what you see in the mirror. There is science behind the importance of it and the role that it plays in our everyday lives.

A great smile is essential to a happy life in today's world.

A simple act of a smile can quite literally transform your world. And I'm not just saying that because I spend my life helping create beautiful smiles. Loving your smile will help you want to show it more. When you use the insider secrets to choose the right dentist for you, you will be on the right path to loving your smile. There's nothing quite like having beautiful teeth and healthy gums.

Choosing the best dentist for you and your family is an important role, and one that you want to put some effort into. The right dentist can make a huge difference when it comes to dreading your appointments or looking forward to them. It can also help set the stage for how your children grow up to feel about going to the dentist. The last thing you want is for your child to fear of going to the dentist and to take that with them into adulthood.

When you choose the right dentist for you and your family, you will be confident in every visit. You will have someone you trust that is putting your best interest first—they hear you, see you, and understand you not only as a patient, but as a person. I know I don't want to be just another number that gets called and serviced. I want to be with professionals who care that I'm there and see me as a person with fears, concerns, wishes, and plans.

So why read this boring little book? While it will help you find the right dentist for you and your family, it is going to do far more for your family beyond that. Having the right dentist is going to help your kids keep from getting bullied, help increase their job success in the future, and keep them feeling confident about who they are in this world. The last thing any parent wants is for their child to look in the mirror and hate what they see. The good news is by choosing the right dentist you have the ability to prevent that from happening.

CHAPTER 2

How to Confidently Choose the Best Dentist for Your Family

Did you know that finding the right dentist for you and your family is not just a cosmetic issue? It's a health issue as well. Misaligned, crooked teeth are equal to significant medical problems. Poorly aligned teeth can produce chronic headaches and migraines, contribute to digestive problems because of poor chewing of foods, make getting a decent night's sleep impossible, and, maybe most dangerous, foster gum disease. Gum disease is connected to diabetes, heart disease, strokes, and dementia, as well as, of course, loss of natural teeth altogether.

When you think about the number of dentists there are to choose from, it's easy to see why it can be a daunting task to choose one. Well, not just one, but the *right* one. Anyone can choose a dentist, but not everyone will do some homework in order to choose the right dentist, and there's a huge difference between the two. Choosing the right dentist for your family is going to set your mind at ease. It's going to help your family to feel comfortable and confident as they go in for their appointments. And if the time arises that they need treatment, they won't run out the door or try to hide to keep it from happening.

There are over 160,000 dentists in the country. Open your local phone book or do a quick Google search and you will without a doubt find many that are in your local area. You have more dentists available to you than you could care to ever want or need. But don't let that overwhelm you. Choosing the right dentist comes down to one thing: confidence.

Confidence, by definition is having faith that you the choice you make will be the right one. I've talked with many parents over the years, and I hear how they fear making the wrong choice. Until they came to my office, they lacked the confidence that it took to make a dentist selection based on something more than just choosing a name. You probably never gave it much thought, but choosing a dentist should be treated like you are hiring someone for a job. In essence, that's exactly what you are doing.

TIME WELL SPENT

There isn't one thing you can do to choose the right dentist for your family. I wish it were that easy, as I'm sure you do as well. Rather, it's a variety of things that you will do in order to help lead you to the right selection. Don't worry, though, I don't want you to think this is a process that is going to be extremely time-intensive. You shouldn't have to spend a great deal of time on these things.

The health implications of making sure you have the right dentist goes further than you may realize. When teeth are not properly cared for, the gums can pull away from the teeth, which allows pockets and the harboring of infection. Periodontal disease turns into a very difficult, painful, and costly problem later in life. Most people don't realize it, but the $4,000 that is not spent during the teen years can easily require a $40,000 full-mouth restoration later in life.

Not only that, but periodontal disease compromises health, and often leads to tooth loss and the need for dentures. Gum disease is serious business. It increases the complications and risks of other diseases, such as diabetes, heart disease, strokes, and dementia. If you ignore caring for preteen or teen teeth, especially if there are misalignments present, you are virtually guaranteeing other health problems later in life.

Yes, it will take some to find the right dentist. But it's going to be time well spent, and will be well worth it in the long run. It can help you and your family avoid many awful diseases, pain, and embarrassment, possibly even helping to avoid earlier death due to some of those diseases. Think about how much time you have spent choosing or going to a dentist who doesn't feel right for you. By putting in a little time to find the right one, you can help avoid the dreaded feeling you get when it's time for the next appointment. You will no longer be sitting in the waiting room wondering if you should have found another dentist prior to that appointment, and when will you ever finally get busy doing it?

The questions will be over, the doubt will be over, and you can stop wishing you had a better dentist, or one that is a better fit for your family. By putting in the time to read this book and doing a little of the recommended legwork, you will walk away with a dentist who is perfect for your family. In the whole scheme of things, this is going to save you a lot of time, headache, doubt, stress, and more.

While there are specific questions you will want to ask the dentists you interview for the job, we will cover those in a later chapter. For now, let's look at some of the other things you can uncover and discover in order to help make you feel confident about choosing the right dentist for your family.

Remember, the time you put into finding the right dentist is an investment in your family's dental health, as well as their psychological well-being and long term. So don't take shortcuts. We want to do what we need to in order to weed out those who are not a good fit and get to the best of the best. Keep in mind that the best of the best for someone else may not be the best of the best for your family. You may have different needs, wants, and goals, and you will need to keep that in mind as you go along.

WHERE TO LOOK

There are many places to look to begin your search for the right dentist, but let's take a look at some of the most popular options. This way we can take a look at the pros and cons of these choices, and narrow down which may be the better routes to consider taking.

You will find that advice and information regarding choosing a dentist abounds. But that doesn't mean you should listen to all of the advice you receive. As with anything else, you should consider the source, take some things with a grain of salt, and still take steps to include researching the candidate. There's nothing that will replace simply doing some good old-fashioned research on the person you are considering hiring as your family dentist.

Some of the most popular ways that people find new dentist leads include:

- Recommendations they may receive from their friends, family members, or co-workers.

- By conducting searches online and reviewing their website, social media pages, or reading reviews about them.

- Through general advertising that you may see online, on a billboard, in a magazine, or on the television.

- Seeing a dentist be featured in a news story, whether on television or in print, or in another type of article or news story.

- Spotting a dentist's office as you are driving near your home, school, or office.

- By looking at the in-network provider list provided by your insurance company.

There may be additional ways that people find their way to a dentist, but these are the most common ways. In order to find the right dentist for your family, you have to start out with knowing where to look for them. Once you have narrowed down a few ideal candidates, you will be ready to move on to taking the step of researching and interviewing them.

Ideally, you will come up with a short list of candidates that you will take the time to evaluate. This is the most effective way to determine the best doctor for you. Sometimes people may look good on paper, but they have a personality that doesn't click with your family. Or perhaps they look a little sterile on paper and in looking at their credentials, but when you meet there is an instant connection with their personality. Their credentials matter a lot, but so does their personality—you want them to fit in well with your family and help you feel comfortable and secure when you go in for every visit.

You want a dentist you not only feel comfortable with, but one you can trust—one you feel will listen to you and your family. Everyone wants to feel heard and that they are cared about, but many dentists are in such a hurry today that they limit their interactions with each patient. If that appeals to you, great, but if it doesn't then you will want to find a dentist who takes the time you need. You want your questions answered, and you want to feel like you are the most important thing for him to focus on when you are in the chair. If the dentist is being pulled in many different directions, you may feel that the distractions are a bit too much and that you are not the center of attention at a time when you should be.

GETTING PERSONAL RECOMMENDATIONS

When you begin looking for dentist recommendations from people you know, you want to narrow down if there is a specific type of dentist you are looking for. While most people have experience with a general dentist, for example, they may not have experience with someone who specializes in cosmetic or pediatric dentistry. If you have a desire or need for a specific type of dentist, then you need to let people know that from the start, so you are not given recommendations to numerous general dentists who do not handle such areas.

It's difficult for people to recommend a specialist dentist if they haven't had experience with the person themselves. When seeking personal recommendations from people, you want to hear the direct experience they have had with the dentist. You are trusting your smile to the dentist you choose, so you want to make sure that you are choosing the right one for your family. Ending up with someone who isn't a good fit will leave you with regrets and possibly not liking your smile. It can also leave your kids growing up with a fear of the dentist that will stick with them for a lifetime.

The dentist your friends and family recommend may be fine for them, or they may not know much about the person either. Your friends likely don't realize the long-term consequences of not having a dentist you can trust and who will guide you in providing the best care for your family's teeth. Remember, there's more at stake here than cosmetics.

Most general dentists will offer cosmetic dentistry, and many of them do see children. But that doesn't mean they are experts on those areas, so if they are of concern to you, be sure that the dentist you choose has expertise in them. Many general dentists will not begin seeing children until they are of a certain age, usually around five or seven or so, but pediatric dentists will begin seeing children at only a year old. And if you are in need of cosmetic dentistry, sedation or implant dentistry, you will want to choose someone who is well experienced with it, so that you get a great return on your investment.

To get recommendations from family, friends, and co-workers, you could post about it on your social media networks, such as Facebook. Let people know the type of dentist you are looking for and give them an idea of location, since those who follow you are likely to cover a large geographic area. From there, you can take it further to ask questions that may come to mind, based off what they said or questions that you may have on your own. Some additional questions to consider for those giving you recommendations include:

- How long have you been going to that dentist and do your family members also love going there?

- Is there any type of specific treatments that the dentist has experience in?

- How experienced is this dentist and how much experience did you personally have with the person?

- When you need treatment, did the dentist explain what options were available to you, along with all of the advantages and disadvantages of them?

- When you had treatment done, how well did the dentist explain to you the procedure, so you knew what to expect? Did they explain to you how long the treatment process would take, and how long things like crowns would last?

- What is the dentist's policy when it comes to guarantees or protecting you if you are not happy with the treatment or if it doesn't hold up as it should?

There is a chance that the person giving you the recommendation doesn't know the answer to all of these questions. Plus, you don't necessarily want to ask them every question and grill them over the recommendations. Pick and choose which follow-up questions make sense for the recommendations you are getting, based off what they said they liked about the dentist and what you feel is appropriate to ask.

If your insurance provider gave you a list of dentists who are in their network, it may give you a referral, but they are only telling you what dentists have contracted with that insurance company to accept discounted fees in return for their patients. It doesn't speak at all about what they specialize in, what their hours are like, how their personality is, or if they will be a good fit for your family.

While it's nice to have a dentist who is part of the preferred network, that approach may not always get you the best dentist for your family. Use the information as a starting point, but if you feel the best dentist for your family is not on the network list, speak to your insurance company to see what arrangements can be made. Costs and insurance play little part in the overall picture and shouldn't be the determining factor in choosing a dentist if you want the best one for your family. Don't let fears about network lists keep you from seeking out the best dentist for your family.

Excellent dentists have some characteristics in common that lend to their great abilities and service. Some of the characteristics of excellent dentists you want to look for include:

- How friendly is the dentist? Is the person caring and attentive to your needs and concerns? Do they take the time to answer your questions thoroughly, so you feel comfortable with the information you have received? Do they explain the procedures so you know what to expect and what the likely outcome will be?

- Does the dentist have the training and experience that you want and need in order to have the treatments done that you desire? How long have they been in practice and what type of experience do they have? Is there anything they specialize in, such as cosmetic or pediatric dentistry?

- How will the dentist handle an emergency situation? What if the emergency happens on the weekend? Will they still see you?

- Does the dentist keep up with the latest technology and techniques? This is important if you are looking for advanced cosmetic dentistry or to help reduce discomfort during treatment.

- How much of a part of your community is the dentist? Do they give back, get involved, and seem to be a part of the community?

- How do they treat new patients in terms of being able to get appointments? Will you be waiting months to have your first appointment?

- What types of things is the dentist able to do in order to help you or someone in your family with anxiety about going to their office?

A great dentist is going to go above and beyond for every patient. Just providing you with the treatment you expected when you walked in the door is not enough. Of course, that's what they should provide, but that is not going to excite you and get you loving that dentist office.

CHILDREN AND BEING NICE

If you have children, you will want to pay extra attention to the recommendations you receive and keep that in mind. Choosing the right dentist for your children is crucial so they have a good foundation. Children who grow up going to a dentist who is not a good fit for them may end up hating or fearing going to the dentist as adults. You can help avoid and alleviate such fears and stress by ensuring they have a child-friendly dentist while they are growing up. Pairing them with the right dentist will help them learn to trust dentists, rather than fear going to them. You want your child to see their dentist as someone who is there to help them, not cause them pain and undue stress, and you can only do that by matching them with the right one.

It's also important to note that you don't want to choose a dentist based on the idea that someone is nice. I once had a patient tell me that they went to a dentist's office where the hygienist was super nice. The woman was soft-spoken, friendly, and super gentle. Almost too nice, if that's even possible. But the problem, as she explained it, was that when she left their office she didn't feel like her teeth were even cleaned. The woman was so mild-mannered and gentle that the patient didn't feel that her teeth got the usual cleaning that she had grown accustomed to. And to make matters worse, because the hygienist was nice, she didn't have the heart to complain about it.

That's not a good situation to get into. Not only will you not be happy with the dental experience you are receiving, but you will also either grow frustrated as time goes on, or you will simply fade away, finding a new dentist office to try. Being nice is great and it is necessary when working with patients, but that should not be the only criteria for which you choose a dentist office. You want nice, but you also want them to know what they are doing, be well experienced, be attentive to your wishes, and make you feel like your time there was well spent. Being nice also doesn't ensure that they specialize in the treatment options you are looking for, so look for nice, but also look beyond it to get the whole package.

Here's what I hear from many patients: "My parents were great, but I wish they would have gotten us a better dentist. Growing up, I was embarrassed of my mouth and would try to not show my smile. I would also cover up my mouth whenever I laughed. I didn't dare want people to see my teeth. Here I am today trying to spend a fortune to fix the problems that resulted from not getting it right to begin with."

We owe it to our family to help them get the best start that they can get. That goes for their teeth, too, since they are such an important part of someone's confidence and play such an important role in their long-term health.

ADVERTISING AND INTERNET REFERRALS

Many dentists engage in advertising their services. There is nothing wrong with using advertising as a starting point in narrowing down your search for a great dentist. It should be a starting point, though, because the ad will not answer all of your questions or let you know if their personality is a good fit for your family.

One thing that advertising should do is answer a few of the questions you have regarding any specialty areas they focus on. Most dentists who advertise will want to let readers know that they do cosmetic dentistry, sedation dentistry, pediatrics, or that they offer weekend appointments. They will want to get those key points into their ad, so they can help you narrow down your search.

If you see an advertisement for a dentist that catches your eye and gets your attention, take the info and do your additional research. You will still want to see if others you know have ever gone to the person and what their experience was like and you will want to be sure to interview the dentist and ask questions.

Today, it's common for people to begin their search for a new dentist online. While there is a ton of information regarding dentists online, there's one word to sum up how you should approach it: caution.

The Internet can be both great and horrible for finding a new dentist. You have immediate access to a plethora of information on the one hand, but on the other, you have no idea how valid any of it is. In today's world, there are people who pay for good reviews to be posted, you can have negative reviews posted by someone who is actually your competition, and you may have people leaving reviews on sites who have never even been near the dentist's office they are leaving a review for. In other words, take what you find online with a grain of salt and still do your in-person evaluation.

As with anything you read online, you have to consider the source. If you are at the dentist's website, you can take what is on there at face value. They are likely to provide you with truthful information about what treatments they provide, the types of payment they accept, and detailed information about the people who will be taking care of you and your family there. If you are not on the dentist's website, pay close attention to the source as to whether or not it's a well-respected site or one that anyone can post anything on a whim. Always consider the source.

In today's high-tech world, there are many review and ranking sites online. People can go there and put in their two cents on everything from their experience at hiring a plumber to staying at a particular hotel. They seem like they could be a great thing, and often times they are if you are looking for a new restaurant to try. That's because trying out a new restaurant isn't a big investment and won't be all that costly. Even if it was a horrible meal you are not out that much, so the loss isn't so great. But take the advice on something as important as a dentist and not be happy with the choice and it could have a much bigger implication for you and your family.

I know wonderful dentists with zero online reviews because they have small practices and do very little advertising. I also know average and below-average dentists who have paid online marketing services for wonderful, fake reviews. Start your online search with the understanding that the information may not be all that accurate. Use it as a starting point, but carry on with the rest of your research just the same.

FEATURED DENTISTS

Chances are you have seen dentists featured in your area either in the news or in articles in newspapers and magazines. This is a great way to be introduced to a dentist, but again, treat it as a starting point. I know many dental professionals who have been featured in articles and news stories and they often have impeccable resumes and a great fan base. But that doesn't mean that every dentist you see on the news is going to be the right one for you.

Some dentists make their way into the media coverage because the reporter has selected them due to their reputation in the local field. Others may be featured because they are an advertiser on the news station or in the publication, so when they need a dental source they are called upon. Still, others may be working with a public relations agency that helped them get that media spot. When a dentist works with a public relations firm, they pay them a fee so that in turn they get media exposure. This is not to say anything bad about public relations work, because it's a great thing and can help dentists get their name into the public. Yet it is good for you to understand the different ways in which some dentists may get media exposure.

Having confidence in choosing the dentist who is right for you and your family starts with having a few candidates to consider. Those candidates who make your short list may come from a variety of places, including personal recommendations from family and friends, or they may come from names you have seen in advertisements or the general media. No matter how you obtain those names that make your short list, keep in mind that they are a starting point. You still have some work to do once you have those names, but I promise you that if you stick with it and see this through, you will be happy with the choice you make.

Confidently choosing the best dentist for your family starts with putting together a short list of candidates that you will further research and evaluate in order to narrow it down to the candidate you select. Simply put, choosing the right dentist for you and your family is too big of an investment to take it lightly. Scouting out the best dentist who is a good fit for your family will help ensure happy smiles, beautiful teeth, comfortable patients, and the end to battles, tears, and fear over dentist appointments.

CHAPTER 3

Relax: We've Got You Covered

Did you know that approximately 25 percent of all students have been bullied in school?[5] It's true. As an adult, you may realize that bullying is nothing new. Heck, we all experienced some kind of bullying and razzing when we were growing up. But things are different today. A lot different.

Today's bullying is no longer classmates teasing you a little bit about this or that. When we were growing up there was some teasing, but today's bullying has taken measures to a whole new level. Kids are committing suicide over what's going on today. Plus, with the emergence of social media, the bullying can be relentless. Years ago, when the kids left the schoolyard, the bullying stopped. Today, since

---

5   "Facts About Bullying," stopbullying.gov, https://www.stopbullying.gov/media/facts/index.html

most kids have cellphones and access to social media, the bullying continues nonstop. Today's bullying has the ability to spread like wildfire.

This brings us to the question of why are most kids bullied in the first place? As the adults in their life, we not only want to know the answer to this question, but we want to do something about it if we can. In recent years, because the bullying issue has become so common and increasingly brutal, researchers have taken to trying to answer exactly that question. What they have found is that most kids are bullied because of their looks.

There are a few key studies that point to the importance of children being bullied in regard to their physical appearance. These are studies that every parent should be aware of so they can try to do what is within their power to help their child overcome this situation.

- In the 2014 issue of the European Journal of Dentistry, researchers reported that facial aesthetics, including oral appearance, could severely affect children's quality of life, causing physical, social, and psychological impairment. They also reported that children and adolescents with aesthetic-related dental malformations are potential targets for bullies. They go on to advise that providing an adequate aesthetic dental treatment is an important step, and they noted the operation lead to significant improvement in self-esteem, self-confidence, socialization, and academic performance of all patients.

- A December 2014 study published in the American Journal of Orthodontics and Dentofacial Orthopedics reported the results of research that was conducted on 920 children in order to see if there was a relationship between bullying and dental issues. What researchers found was there was a significant relationship between bullying and dentofacial features, indicating a negative effect on oral health-related quality of life.

- In the May 2016 issue of the journal *Crisis*, researchers shared the results of a study that was conducted to examine whether experiences of verbal abuse, physical abuse, and cyberbullying were uniquely associated with a general suicide risk. Their results showed that all types of bullying were associated with a suicide risk.

The important takeaways here are that bullying is happening now more than ever. Kids who have oral issues are at an increased risk for being the target of bullying, and all types of bullying is associated with a suicide risk. This is a disheartening issue that every parent needs to be aware of. Your family's dental care is significantly linked to their overall well-being in life.

But don't think that it's only children who you need to be concerned with when it comes to choosing the right dentist. You and other adults in your home are affected as well. The World Health Organization reports: "Oral health affects people physically and psychologically and influences how they grow, enjoy life, look, speak, chew, taste food and socialize, as well as their feelings of social well-being."

As you can see, oral health is a major contributing factor in how happy our lives are and contributes to us actually enjoying them. It's too important of an issue to not find the right dentist for you and your family.

AVOIDING THE DENTIST

I've talked with many patients over the years who will share with me that they hadn't been to a dentist in a while. For some of them, it had been years. There's a pattern with many people who actively try to avoid the dentist—they may only make an appointment when they have an issue that they can no longer tolerate. They find themselves in terrible pain or discomfort, the medicines they are trying are no longer helping, and they simply can't take it any longer. That's when they make an appointment with the dentist. Yet, if they had been going all along, there's a chance that pain and discomfort would have been avoided in the first place.

So, what is it that makes people avoid going to the dentist in the first place? They do this despite knowing that it's so much better for them to go, and not all that time consuming. In all honesty, those who keep up with regular dental visits are likely to go only twice per year, and be there for probably an hour each time. That's not a lot of time to put into taking professional care of one's teeth, considering all that oral health impacts.

Let's look at some of the reasons why people don't go to the dentist, or they try to put it off as long as they can.

TIME

Many people believe they will have to miss school or work in order to fit in dental appointments. While it's true that at one time, dentists pretty much only kept banker hours, that's not the case today. An important part of finding the right dentist for you is finding one who offers appointment hours that are comfortable for you. In my practice, we offer early morning appointments—great for our busy patients!

FEAR

Let's be honest here. Many, many people fear the dentist. They may recall when they were kids how there were painful procedures involved in going to the dentist. Many people are fearful that the dentist will judge or shame them. They may also have this fear from listening to stories from other people, or by watching movies that have made doing to the dentist look like a painful experience. Mention something like a root canal and many people will wince, reinforcing the myth that it's a super painful experience. Let's put these fears to rest right here and now. Technology has come a long, long way. Going to the dentist today and having treatments done is painless. Most people don't feel the shots anymore that numb their mouth, sedation is an option, and tools have been designed to provide more comfort during every procedure. What hurts more is not going to have the treatments done that are needed. Not only will avoiding necessary procedures lead to physical problems, but you have already read about all of the emotional pain it can create as well. In today's modern dental world, people should have far more fear about not going to the dentist than they ever do for going.

COSTS

There are a lot of people who avoid going to the dentist because they feel like it's going to be equivalent to taking on a second mortgage. Sure, it can cost some money going to the dentist. There's no doubt about that. But often times that happens because people didn't keep up with dental appointments, which allows costly problems to be created. However, it is important to keep in mind that whatever the cost, the investment you make in your teeth is an investment you make in yourself. That's exactly what getting regular oral care is all about, as is finding the right dentist for you and your family. It's an investment in you and in your family.

But let's look at the costs a little more to determine if it really is something to be feared so much that it should keep people away. It's estimated that the average cost of teeth cleaning around the country is around $98 for adults and $87 for children. Keep up with that and do it twice per year and you are not spending much money, and it can help save you thousands in the long run (not to mention the emotional costs it is saving). That's if you pay cash out of pocket, but many people have dental benefits that are available to everyone at low yearly premiums, which may make it as low as $20–$30 out of pocket for each cleaning. There's nothing expensive about that. Plus, if you have insurance you will find that it can either cover much of the cost of treatment or it will give you a significant discount. If, by chance, someone does need a treatment that is costly, there are typically options to help, such as payment plans and financing. Again, this is still an investment in yourself that will be well worth the cost.

DENTAL ANXIETY

There are some people who have a true anxiety about going to the dentist. It's a condition where they may become so nervous that they can begin to feel sick and stressed out. If you are someone who has such anxiety, speak with the dentist and let them know this. The only way they can help to alleviate the anxiety is to know that you have it. It's estimated that up to 15 percent—or about 48 million—of Americans who avoid the dentist do so because they have a phobia or anxiety toward going. The problem is that if you give in to the anxiety or phobia and avoid going to the dentist, then you will have an increased risk of having oral health problems. Plus, you will have an increased risk of having the many physical and emotional problems that come from not going. The dentist should be able to help you overcome the anxiety and phobia. The right dentist for you will be someone who understands these conditions and is patient enough to help you work through them.

These are just some of the most common reasons that people avoid going to the dentist. Some people avoid going to the dentist because they know they need work done. But that doesn't make a lot of sense when you consider the fact that putting it off is going to make whatever issue the person has even worse, most likely leading them to need even more work.

There are others as well, including the fact that some people may just be lazy. When it comes down to it, they know the importance of it, the health benefits and long term implications of avoiding going, but they just don't make it a priority. While they may mean to go, they put it off and put it off, and before you know it, two years have gone by.

We had a patient in our office who fit that exact category: a well-educated woman who had no fears of going to the dentist. She knew how important it was, but she didn't like the current dentist she had. So the conversation went a little something like this:

"I'm embarrassed to say it's been about three and half years since I had my teeth cleaned."

"Why is that?" we asked her.

"Time just got by me, I guess. I used to always go religiously, but then I moved and didn't act quickly to find a new dentist office. It was always in the back of my mind, but I just didn't get it done."

Don't put it off. Finding the right dentist is far too important to let it rest on the back burner. Make it a priority.

WE'RE HERE FOR YOU

By now you are probably feeling a bit overwhelmed at all that can happen if you don't happen to find the right dentist for your family. That's understandable, considering all that is at stake, but have no fear. You can relax, because we really do have you covered. The information you are getting in this book is invaluable to helping you be able to not only understand the importance of selecting the best dentist for your family, but in determining how to do it.

We are able to give you this information because we know. We've been there. While we are on the dental professional side, we know what it's like on the other side, too. We've done the research, talked to many patients over the years, and seen what happens when you do find the right dentist, as well as when you don't. Our careers have become our passion and we have taken the liberty to study it, learning everything we can about the need for excellent dental care.

When it comes down to it, you want a dentist office that is going to remember your birthday, be involved in the community, and remember who you are by name. When you sit down in their chair, you want them to remember that you are passionate about the Dodgers, or whatever your thing is, and you want them to ask you about it. You want them to surprise you with thank you notes and for them to show gratitude that out of all the dentist offices in the area, you chose their office.

If your dentist doesn't do all of that, and most of them don't, then you are not with the right dentist. The right dentist will make you feel appreciated and that you are their only patient that day. They will give you the time you deserve so that you understand everything, make sure all of your questions are answered, and that you feel confident and comfortable with everything that takes place.

Everyone deserves a dentist who is going to provide them with well above average care. Anyone can provide you with average care, but you should want more than that and seek out more than that. Remember the days when you used to pull up to a gas pump and someone came to your window to see what type of service you wanted? They would wash your windows, check the air in your tire, pump your gas, and more. It was full service. Today, it's pretty much unheard of for someone to get full service like that not only in the gas industry, but pretty much anywhere.

Now imagine what it would be like for you to get full service at the dentist office. From the moment you step into the door you feel special; the people working there are attentive to your needs. They show appreciation for you being there, they make you feel comfortable. The waiting room is decked out in comfortable furniture, as well as some drinks for your wait. When you get called back to the room, the dentist is happy to see you, and speaks to you as if you are old friends. When your birthday rolls around, you get a hand-written birthday greeting in the mail. What would such full service at the dentist office feel like? It would feel amazing, and believe me, it's out there. Full service is what we offer, because we have you covered.

BEDSIDE MANNER ABOVE ALL

Years ago, people felt that they had a better connection with their dentists and other doctors. Bedside manner, as it was referred to, was something that was at the top of the priority list for every person looking for a new dentist. Bedside manner in a nutshell is the approach that the dentist, or any other doctor, takes in their attitude toward the patient.

Bedside manner has largely become an issue most people don't speak about today, but it's something that everyone feels. Patients feel the attitude that the dentist has toward them, whether it is one of indifference or one of gratitude. They can be caring, or they can be callous and not engaged. Whether you call it bedside manner or dental chair side manner, it's still important today.

Find a dentist who has a great chairside manner and you will find that you get much more out of the relationship. You will feel like you have a connection to the dentist, and that connection is important to feeling comfortable, confident, and knowing you have the right dentist for you and your family.

Not having the right dentist for your family can be a scary thing. It can make people want to avoid the dentist and they may not get the best care even if they do go for appointments. Choosing the best dentist for your family is going to make a world of difference in your smiles, but as well as with your emotional well-being. Your teeth are an investment in you, now and well into the future.

CHAPTER 4

Why Is Your Smile So Important?

Have you ever thought about what you may be missing out on if you don't like your smile? What about those people who dislike their smile so much that they hide it when they laugh, or they refuse to show their teeth when they smile? What is that doing to their mental health? You may be surprised at just how much a smile is linked to when it comes to our emotional well-being and our quality of life overall.

There is actually a lot of information out there about how important a smile is. Let's take a child's grades in school, for example. There's a good chance that most people don't even think about the fact that there is a connection between their child's grades and how they feel about their smile. If they bring home good grades it will sure make you smile, but are there things happening in school that are keeping them from smiling, and ultimately from getting better grades?

A child's grades are absolutely linked to how they feel about themselves. Most kids want to get good grades. It's rare that a child sets out to get poor grades or not do well in school. They want the positive reinforcement of getting good grades and making their parents and teachers happy. But often times there are things going on at school that affect their ability to achieve the level of success that they would like to. Some kids may know exactly why they fall behind, while others may feel like a hamster on a wheel—trying hard only to find out each reporting period that they are not really going anywhere.

There isn't just one thing that goes into helping kids get good grades. There are numerous things that all work together to help make it happen. These include things like regular attendance, daily recess when as an elementary student, proper sleep, being prepared, and having parents who are involved. But there are some other equally important factors that contribute to their getting good grades, including:

- **Bullying**. Unfortunately, bullying has become all too common in schools around the country. Along with taking place during the school day, bullying even follows kids home, with them being cyberbullied online or through texting. Not only does this lead them to having a poor self-image, but according to the American Psychological Association, it may also contribute to lower test scores. They believe this may be due to the fact that bullied students often become less engaged in learning. Parents can help tackle this issue by finding out if their child is bullied (oftentimes kids don't tell their parents they are being bullied) and then taking measures to help stop it.

- **Self-image**. How children view themselves plays a big role in how successful they will be academically. Kids who feel good about themselves, including the way they look and their abilities, will likely do better academically. In the September 2016 issue of *Annals of the New York Academy of Sciences*, researchers reported that academic self-efficacy was the most robust predictor of academic achievement. In other words, how they feel about themselves and their abilities is paramount. If they feel good and believe they can achieve their goals and get good grades, then they arc far more likely to do so. To help in this area, parents can help their kids to have a healthy self-image and do things to ensure they are confident.

It stands to reason that if your child doesn't like the way they look that it will have a negative impact on their grades. They will not want to get as involved with others, they will shy away in the classroom, avoid doing presentations, and may be bullied more. There is so much at stake when it comes to a child liking their teeth and smile that we as the adults in their life have to do what we can to help them in this area. Not liking the shape of their feet is one thing that we may not be able to do anything about, but ensuring that their teeth are well taken care of so that they like the way they look is well within our power.

Helping children love their teeth and smile should be a priority of every parent, because there's so much in life that is connected to how they feel about it.

JOBS MATTER, TOO

Loving your smile, and helping your kids to love theirs, doesn't just have an impact on how everyone feels about their grades. It sticks with them and can have an influence over many other areas in their life. Those who don't like the way they look usually have lower self-esteem, and when that happens they will go to job interviews giving off those vibes.

Having low self-esteem tends to make people seem that they lack the confidence to get the job done. Those who don't feel confident tend to let it show through their body language, which is something that people immediately pick up on. Not liking your smile can also have a negative impact on your job and career, because you are less likely to speak up, get involved, close the deal, and take the necessary career risks that can lead you to the next level.

Those with low self-esteem on the job will also lack the confidence to ask for a raise or negotiate a higher salary right from the start. As you can see, not loving your teeth is costing you; it's costing you a lot. Those who fear the costs of investing in their smile should consider the high cost of not investing in their smile.

Self-image is extremely important in most areas of our life. How we feel about ourselves has an impact on our interpersonal relationships, schoolwork, peer relationships, careers, and more. Something as small as a great smile can have a major impact on many areas of your life. It is imperative that you choose the right dentist for your family. Too much is at stake not to.

Liking your smile is not something beyond your reach, and it's something that everyone deserves. When you like your teeth and smile, you are going to have a much better time in life, be happier, and will be putting your best foot forward when it comes to helping your child get better grades and helping them get a good start in the adult future. You will be helping yourself to improve your quality of life, further your career, and make better connections with those around you.

THE SCIENCE BEHIND A SMILE

Now that you know the impact that a great smile has on everything from grades to being bullied and not getting hired for a job, let's dig a little deeper. There is a lot of science behind how important a great smile is in one's life, too. There's a lot that goes on behind the scenes when it comes to smiles, and it's something that most people never even consider.

Have you ever noticed that when you smile at people they tend to smile back? Smiles can be contagious. People smile, which leads to more people smiling, a happier community, and a nicer place to live.

Smiling affects your brain, your attitude, and the way people respond to you. It's part of body language, which is essential to communication overall as we do most of our communicating with our body language. It's amazing how well woven into our life a smile really is and the impact that it has on us.

Internally, there is something incredible that happens with a simple smile. When you smile, it helps to relieve stress, because your brain releases what are called neuropeptides (feel-good transmitters that are released like endorphins, serotonin, and dopamine). One quick smile on your face, and your brain immediately goes into action releasing these feel-good chemicals into your body that make you happy.

Did you know that you don't have to actually be happy for the smile to have this impact? You can force the smile and have it lead to happiness, rather than the other way around. The next time you feel down, force yourself to hold a smile on your face for about two minutes. Sure, it's a fake smile that you are forcing, but here's the thing: Your brain doesn't realize that. Your brain gets the signal that there is a smile on your face and begins pumping out the feel-good chemicals. Next thing you know, your mood is lifted, you feel better, and your stress level has diminished.

In other words, when it comes to smiling, you can fake it until you make it. The endorphins that are released by your brain when you are smiling act as a natural pain reliever in your body. The serotonin works to lift your mood so that you don't feel sad or depressed, serving as a natural built-in antidepressant. Consider how many people take prescription pain pills and antidepressants every year. Smiling more can help keep pain and depression away, as well as help people avoid these costly drugs that have potentially harmful side effects.

Since smiling releases these important feel-good chemicals in the body, it can help to transform your life and the lives of those around you. When you feel happier, you are going to be in a better mood, helping to improve their quality of life and add to their happiness. So much is tied to the smile, yet so many people let time go by without putting one on their face.

Smiling is what is considered an active expression. It's one that draws people in and engages others. Think about it: When is the last time you saw someone with a pinch-faced look or an angry face and it made you want to engage with that person? Most likely not often, because if you see someone like that, your initial reaction is going to be to head the other direction or avoid engaging them. But if you see someone smiling, that active expression is more inviting and there is a good chance you will engage. You will smile back, say a few words, or just make friendly eye contact.

People are drawn toward those who have friendly faces and who are smiling. The more you like your smile and teeth, the more likely you are to have a smile on your face more often. This is going to make you feel more comfortable interacting with others. Smiling helps you connect with others in a happy and positive manner, and that's something we can all use. Showing a beautiful smile and teeth makes you look friendlier, more relaxed, happier, and more approachable to those around you. This goes for you, as well as your children, who are at a vulnerable period for making friends and connecting with others.

THERE'S EVEN MORE SCIENCE

Researchers tend to do studies on a broad range of topics each year, but it's no surprise that they have done so much on the act of smiling. Even before we had the scientific proof to back it up, we all kind of knew the importance of a smile and how it can impact your life. We have all felt and seen it, and it's something that is universal. Even if you don't understand someone else's language, a smile is something we can all understand. We know that it's a friendly gesture that is meant to show a good nature.

When endorphins are released when we smile it makes us feel happier, but it also helps to relieve stress. We know that stress in our body can lead to some major health issues, such as cardiovascular disease. The cortisol in our body is active when we feel stressed or anxious, but it's combated when the endorphins are released from smiling. Smiling is actually good for your overall health, too.

We also know that laughing is good for us, even improving the body's homeostasis. The first step to laughing is a good old-fashioned smile. You can't laugh without smiling. Laughing brings oxygen into the body, releases stress and tension, and helps keep us healthy. Laughing also helps us to release emotions, so if you have something on your mind that is causing distress, you can have a good laugh and that will all ease away.

Smiling not only lifts your mood and helps you to be a happier person, but it helps to improve your immune system. A smile literally creates chemical changes within the body that strengthen your immune system, thus helping to keep you from getting sick and being able to fight off viruses quicker. Doctors have even seen the power of a smile when they take someone's blood pressure. Smiling before getting blood pressure taken helps to lower the rate and give you a better reading.

Finally, it's important to state one of the obvious reasons that a smile is so important, and that's because it makes us more attractive. People tend to look younger, friendlier, and more attractive when they smile. But there is one caveat here, which is that having great teeth kicks it up a notch. Those who smile and have obvious teeth problems won't shine as being as attractive as they would if they had great teeth. Beautiful people all have one thing in common: a beautiful smile.

Although there is a lot of science and research that tells us about the inner workings and mechanics of a smile, all of these things solidify what we already feel. They let us know a smile is a major component to living a happy life, and that it does great things for us both internally and externally. But we already know intrinsically how important a smile is. This is because it's something we live. When you look in the mirror and smile or you see someone else smiling, you already know the importance that has in your life. You don't need a scientist to tell you that it's good for you, because you can feel that it's good for you. It's nice to have research back up what we know, but in all honesty, it's not telling us anything that we don't already feel and see for ourselves.

Dale Carnegie, writer of the famous book, *How to Win Friends and Influence People*, also knew about the importance of a smile. He knew that smiling is an important part to both winning friends and being able to have the power to influence people. One of the things he said about the importance of a smile was: "A smile costs nothing, but creates much. It enriches those who receive, without impoverishing those who give. It happens in a flash and the memory of it sometimes lasts forever."

Dean Martin hit the nail on the head when he said that when you smile, the whole world smiles with you. That's one of the best ways to look at it. Do you want the world smiling with you? Then you need to smile more, and to smile more you have to love your smile. One of the most effective ways for you and your family members to love their smile is to make sure you choose the right dentist for your family.

Having clean, healthy, and straight teeth gives you and your children the confidence to stop hiding your smile. You may be surprised what your kids will tell me while they are sitting in my chair that they won't tell you while sitting at the dinner table. A straight, clean, and healthy smile can not only give your child the confidence they need to embrace their true worth, but it can also pave the way toward easier socialization at school, social gatherings, in groups, and during extracurricular activities.

Some children may need more than simply getting a yearly checkup and having their teeth cleaned. Those children who have crooked teeth or misalignments not only suffer from additional bullying and a lack of confidence, but it can be a true health issue. They may experience such things as headaches, dry mouth, snoring, drooling, bad breath, and insomnia. All of these can be symptoms they experience from not having straight teeth. It's an issue that is not only uncomfortable because of the way it looks, but also because of the way it physically feels for them.

PEACE OF MIND

One of the most important reasons for helping to ensure your family members have a smile that they like is peace of mind. Without a doubt, you want the best for everyone in your family, or you wouldn't be reading this book to begin with. No parent wants their child to suffer, especially from teeth that hurt, embarrass them, or cause social problems. But the fact is that their formative years are some of the most important ones for their development now and into adulthood.

Ensuring that you choose the right dentist helps you give your family the very best foundation for a great smile. As you know, a smile is so important to our development, our success, and our quality of life. The number one thing we all want in life is happiness, and you cannot have that without a smile.

Giving your kids, and yourself, a great smile by having the best possible dentist for your family, is a gift. It's a gift that will help them in many ways, physically and emotionally.

A great smile is the foundation of a happy life, and brings peace of mind.

CHAPTER 5

Is a Great Smile Just a Cosmetic Issue?

Not having a great smile can lead to bullying, poor grades, and certainly a poorer self-image. A poor smile (and self-image) will keep doors from opening in school, jobs, and relationships. We have already established the many problems that can arise when someone doesn't have a great smile. In order to be successful in life, you need to feel good about the way you look, and liking your smile is a huge part of that.

Not having a great smile can lead to everything from missed job opportunities and lower salaries to not cultivating great interpersonal relationships. When you think about all the damage that can be done to someone's emotional well-being simply because they don't like their smile or teeth, it's clear to see how important the topic is.

But is a great smile just a cosmetic issue? Is there more to the story than what meets the eye with every smile? There's a lot more at stake here than just the cosmetic issue. The cosmetic issue alone is a major area of concern, as I've been sharing in the previous chapters. There is no mistaking how essential it is that people like their teeth and their smile. Going beyond cosmetics, there are plenty of other reasons to make sure that your teeth and smile are great.

The question of oral health is more than just cosmetic, as it relates to your overall physical health, just as well. Poorly aligned teeth can produce chronic headaches, digestive problems due to poor chewing of foods, sleep disorders, and, maybe most dangerous, foster gum disease. Gum disease has absolute links to diabetes, heart disease, strokes and dementia, as well as, of course, loss of natural teeth altogether. Corrections later in adult life are more difficult, can be painful, require time off work, and at best, can be an embarrassment.

Uncorrected mouth problems and misaligned teeth make for strangely stretched gums inevitably destined to separate from teeth and allow pockets for infections and periodontal disease that turns into very difficult, painful, and costly problems late in life.

Not spending $4,000 in the teens can easily create a $40,000 full mouth restoration case at age forty or fifty, or an embarrassing, health-compromising removal of all teeth and use of dentures at age sixty. Certainly there is no better time to tackle your problems, than right now!

Gum disease is serious business. It worsens risks of and heightens dangers from diabetes, heart disease, strokes, and dementia. Ignore teeth misalignment and you virtually guarantee adult medical problems. If there is genetic history of any of these medical problems I just named, you only worsen the odds of your children suffering from them by ignoring or just postponing needed orthodontic treatment.

Perhaps you are thinking that nobody in your family needs braces, and it appears as though you all have straight teeth without any problems to worry about. Okay, while I can't say for sure because I haven't done an examination to see if there are underlying issues that need to be corrected, for the sake of this discussion we will go with it. Well, tooth alignment treatment aside, there are still many reasons why having a great dentist is crucial to your overall health. Let's start by talking about periodontal disease.

NASTY PERIODONTAL DISEASE

If you haven't heard it before, let me be the first to tell you that periodontal disease is nasty. And you and your family members do not want it. In fact, you want to stay as far away from it as possible. The more you learn about it, the more likely are to agree that it's something you want to steer clear of now and long into the future.

Periodontal disease is typically what results from inflammation and infections that take place in the gums and the bones that surround the teeth. In the early stages of periodontal disease, it starts out as gingivitis. During this state, the gums become inflamed and red, as well as swollen. You may also find that they bleed when you brush your teeth. Left untreated, gingivitis will continue to advance, wreaking havoc on your mouth.

When you have gingivitis that is allowed to advance, it can end up making your gums pull away from the teeth. That is simply nothing to mess with. What do you think happens when the gums pull away from the teeth? Well, the gums are a big part of what is holding the teeth in your mouth, so when they pull away you risk losing teeth.

With gingivitis, you begin to see the destruction just getting started. The redness, inflammation, and bleeding gums are huge signs there is a problem that needs to be addressed immediately. Left untreated, it continues to advance and move into a stage called periodontitis. It's in this stage that the gums pull away from the teeth. This causes the teeth to loosen and possibly fall out.

One of the biggest threats to your oral health is periodontal disease.

Without consistent dental care, gum disease can easily creep in when you least expect it. According to the Centers for Disease Control and Prevention, just over 47 percent of all adults who are over the age of thirty have some form of periodontal disease.

Think about it for a moment: nearly half of all adults in the country are walking around with a disease that can lead to their gums bleeding, pulling away from their teeth, and potential tooth loss. This is serious stuff. And it doesn't get better; the stats actually get worse as you age. By the time adults reach the age of sixty-five, 70 percent of them have periodontal disease.

Here are a few more statistics from the American College of Prosthodontists that show you just how important of an issue taking care of your teeth is:

- More than 36 million Americans don't have any teeth. There are *36 million* people in this country who don't have any teeth at all.

- Tooth loss happens from decay and gum disease, which can be a result of wear, cancer, injury, etc.

- Of those who have no teeth, around 90 percent of them have dentures.

- They estimate that the problem of toothlessness will continue to grow to more than 200 million people within the next fifteen years.

It may seem as though it's a simple issue. When you lose teeth, you just go get dentures. But it's not that simple. There are some serious health problems that can arise from having missing teeth, which many people find surprising.

Some of the consequences of missing teeth can include nutritional changes, some forms of cancer, coronary artery disease, and obesity. These are serious problems that can arise from missing teeth, so it's imperative to try to take the best possible care of your teeth throughout your life—including finding the right dentist for you and your family and then visiting regularly for check-ups and any necessary treatments that are recommended to you.

In a 2013 study that was published in the *International Journal of Dentistry*, researchers explained the connection between oral health and a person's overall general health. In their report, they stated that despite there being advances in preventative dentistry, people losing their teeth (called edentulism) was still a major worldwide health problem.

Some of the key findings from their important study include:

- Edentulism is both debilitating and irreversible. Once someone loses their adult teeth, they cannot reverse that and go back.

- They report that edentulism is more popular among women.

- Studies show that denture wearing continues to increase.

When it comes to how tooth loss impacts overall general health, the researchers report that tooth loss was also associated with eating an unhealthy diet, increased rates of chronic inflammatory changes of the gastric mucosa, and higher rates of peptic ulcers. Those who are missing their teeth also have higher rates of diabetes mellitus, hypertension, heart failure, stroke, sleep apnea, and chronic kidney disease. Furthermore, tooth loss was also associated with a decrease in being physically active and leading a healthy quality of life.

That's an incredible amount of problems that can arise from not taking the best possible care of your teeth. Sure, some of these problems may happen anyway, even if you do try to take good care of your teeth. But by having the best possible dentist, going for regular appointments, and getting treatments as they are needed, you will be doing a great deal to help lower those risks.

Far too often, we go through life not discussing the implications of some of the decisions we make. There are millions of people who don't realize how important their teeth are and the best possible way to care for them until it's too late.

Don't be one of those people. Stop at nothing short of your family having the best possible dentist, who will help you reduce the risks of problems, recommend treatments that are necessary, and will help you continue to have a higher quality of life. Our teeth play a major role in our lives. They may be small, but their impact is tremendous. Taking care of them and finding the best dentist for our family is paramount.

TOOTH DECAY

There's another little area that we need to talk about when it comes to tooth care beyond the cosmetics. That's the area of tooth decay. There's no doubt that you are likely familiar with what cavities are. They are holes in the teeth. But did you know that cavities start from tooth decay? A cavity isn't something that happens overnight. Rather, it is a process that takes place little by little over time.

The good news here is that tooth decay can be stopped, as well as reversed. This will help keep you and your family from getting cavities. But if regular dental visits are not being kept up, then tooth decay is allowed to continue getting worse until one day your child has a tooth that keeps hurting, you take them to a dentist and find out that they have a cavity. Next, you are crossing your fingers that the cavity was found in a state small enough that you can get away with just filling it, rather than needing something more, such as a root canal or crown.

The longer tooth decay is left unaddressed, the more damage it does. The longer cavities are left untreated the more damage they do, and the more it will cost you to repair it. Plus, you can't reverse a cavity. Once the hole is there, it's there forever and you can only do something to fill or cover it. Tooth decay caught early can be addressed and the teeth can be better protected from reaching the state of having a cavity.

It's estimated that 25 percent of the adult population in the country has untreated tooth decay. Consider that for a moment, one out of every four adults who are reading this book is doing so with untreated tooth decay. You may not even be aware that you have it, but it's there, lurking in your mouth, just waiting to wreak havoc on your teeth. Unless you take action to find the best dentist and start getting treatment for that tooth decay, your future will have cavities in it, as well as possibly crowns, root canals, and even tooth loss.

Our mouths are filled with bacteria, and some of it can be harmful to the teeth. If you drink a lot of drinks with sugar in them, or if you eat a lot of starchy foods (cookies, crackers, chips), those create a plaque on the teeth that will lead to mineral loss and tooth decay. The bacteria in your mouth use the sugar and starches to produce acid that eats away at the teeth, starting the downward spiral.

When teeth are repeatedly exposed to the acid attacks, the enamel will continue to lose minerals. Over time, more minerals are lost, and the enamel becomes weak and a hole is created, which is the cavity. Don't let this happen to you and your family, because it can be prevented and reversed.

When the acid that is produced attacks your teeth, it's bad news. That's where you will begin to have tooth decay that can lead to something even worse. That is unless you are seeing a great dentist so that they can help you address it, and reverse the process. Tooth decay can absolutely be treated, but time is of the essence. Getting it addressed immediately is the only way to help ensure that it doesn't spread deeper into the teeth. Left untreated or ignored, the damage will continue to mount.

MAKES A GREAT WINDOW

Many health professionals believe that your oral health is literally a window to your overall health. People who have poor oral health are at a higher risk for having poor health in other areas. We've discussed some of them, but here's a quick rundown of some of the issues that poor oral health is believed to contribute to:

- **Cardiovascular disease**—oral inflammation is believed to increase risks of heart attack and stroke.

- **Premature birth and low birth weight**—it's estimated that around 18 percent of preterm births and low birth weight babies are attributed to mothers having oral infections.

- **Poorly controlled diabetes**—poor oral health may make it more difficult to control diabetes.

Periodontitis has been linked to numerous health problems and diseases. The saliva in your mouth is like a fingerprint. It's that important and can be useful in gathering information about your overall health, as well as for drug testing, hormonal changes, and to test for various diseases. Our mouths and oral health can reveal so much about us, and really does make a great window to our overall health.

Research shows that bacteria associated with gum disease can increase inflammation and raise cholesterol levels. The bacteria can also travel from the mouth to the liver, lungs, kidneys, and heart. This is something that we don't think much about, but it can have a huge impact on our lives and our overall health.

Many people who already have health problems may also be more prone to oral health issues. Certain prescriptions can negatively impact oral health by reducing the amount of saliva that is produced. Some of the disease that can contribute to oral health problems include: diabetes, HIV/AIDS, osteoporosis, eating disorders, rheumatoid arthritis, neck and head cancers, and Alzheimer's disease.

Anyone trying to maintain good overall health should never overlook oral health. The links between the two are profound and the research has shown the many connections. It's important to make sure that you and your family receive the best possible dental care so that you can help to lower the risks of getting a wide variety of diseases over time. People who are on a quest to be healthy often overlook oral health. They tend to start exercising and go on a diet, but they remain unaware of the strong connection between their oral health and their general health overall. Armed with this information, you can use it to help keep you and your family much healthier.

NOT MERELY COSMETIC

As you can see after reading this chapter, a great smile is not just a cosmetic issue. Not by a long shot. In fact, it would be difficult to say which is more important, the psychological health that comes from a great smile, or the overall general health that comes from it. You need both in order to live a well-balanced life that is considered high quality. If you have one without the other you, will be missing out on a lot in your life.

Having a great smile is so much more than just loving what you see in the mirror or in pictures. It's also about the things we can't see with the naked eye, such as what the bacteria in our mouths are doing and how they are impacting the rest of our body. Take care of your oral health and you will be doing a lot of good in helping to take care of your overall health.

With your oral health being such a significant contributor to your overall health and quality of life, it's imperative that you find the right dentist for your family. The right dentist will be an ally, armed with the tools and knowledge you need on your side, to help keep you and your family healthier.

CHAPTER 6

Why Not Just Any Dentist?

What a wonderful world it would be if we could all just trust the fact that any dentist we called up to make an appointment with was a great one. Then we wouldn't have to worry about anything happening that we hadn't bargained for when we made the decision to sit down in their chair. Unfortunately, that's not the world that we live in, and it's likely never going to be.

Believe it or not, not all dentists are the same. Some dentists are satisfied with where they are at in their training when they leave dental school. They may just take enough continuing education to maintain their dental license. Other dentists are always striving to improve their skills and offer more ranges of services to their patients.

The last thing you want is to have made an appointment with a dentist that you regret. As an adult, you may be a little more understanding in that if you go to a dentist who isn't a good fit, you can move on to find another one. But kids are not so easily forgiving in this regard. If you take your child to a dentist who is a lousy fit, you could be setting them up to never want to go to a dentist again. They may immediately form the opinion that it's scary, painful, and something to be avoided at all costs.

Right now, you are helping to lay the foundation for how your children will go through their life addressing their oral care. Several years back, I had a conversation with a man who was around forty years old, and needed something done to one of his teeth because he was in pain. He was the type of person who had been largely avoiding the dentist his entire adult life, only finally breaking down to go in when there was something bothering him to the point that he couldn't take it anymore.

We discussed why it is that he doesn't go to the dentist regularly. He was an intelligent man who understands the importance of good oral care. He realizes that it's important to go to the dentist regularly, so it didn't make a lot of sense why he wasn't going. And this was the example he was setting for his children, who see how often Dad goes to the dentist (or doesn't in this case). So I dug a little deeper to inquire as to why he isn't going regularly, despite him knowing the importance of it. Then he explained and it all made a whole lot of sense.

When this man was a child, he grew up poor and on welfare. His parents took him to the health department of a major city for the dental work that he needed. He wasn't taken there regularly or for teeth cleanings, but typically only when there was a problem. When he was a teenager he recalls the how the dentist made him feel so bad, because he sat there saying things to him like "I can't believe what a mess your teeth are, you have so many problems." The dentist went on and on saying things to him like this, essentially shaming him, yet he was in the office seeking help.

The shame and humiliation this man felt as a young teen laid the groundwork for the relationship he has with dentists today. First of all, he's ashamed to go to the dentist. He feels as though instead of the dentist helping him by providing treatment and being on his side, that he is judging him and is disgusted with his teeth. Secondly, when he was growing up he was only taken to the dentist when there was a problem, so he continues that path today. He was taught you finally break down and go to the dentist, only when you have a problem or pain that persists.

This man doesn't know what it's like to go in for a routine check-up or cleaning. He has been conditioned to think that the dentist is going to humiliate him because he doesn't have great teeth, and that he only needs to go to him as a last resort because the pain or problem won't go away. This is a sad, sad, situation that not only impacts him, but it impacts others, because there is a good chance that his children will grow up to follow in their dad's footsteps. This man's father may have even had the same relationship with dentists while he was growing up, and the cycle continues.

His poor relationship today is a result of what happened to him at the dentist office while he was growing up. While the individual problems may vary, this type of story is repeated among adults around the country. You wouldn't believe how many adults are fearful of the dentist, distrust them, or avoid them, because of the experiences that they had starting out as children.

FIRST IMPRESSIONS MATTER

We all know in life how important first impressions are. We want to believe that we don't judge things from first impressions and in such a quick manner, but the truth of the matter is that our brains are hardwired to do so. Our brains are hardwired to make immediate judgment calls on something and file the information away about whether it was something good, bad, etc. This goes back to our early ancestors, when our brains had to immediately help us to decipher mortal danger. Being able to make immediate judgment calls helped to save our lives. It told us whether we needed to act on our fight or flight instincts.

Imagine for a moment how different things would have turned out for the man I was speaking about if he had gone to a dentist who would have made a better impression on him. What if the dentist would have been more professional, had a better attitude, and looked out for the best interest of this child? Even if the child had sat in his chair and when he peered into his mouth what he saw was a cause for alarm, things could have turned out differently if the dentist had been more professional. What if he had been gentler with him, helped him to not feel ashamed, and led him to believe that the dentist was on his side, that he was going be with him as a united front to treat and help him get to a point where he loved his teeth?

What an incredible difference this dentist would have made in that young person's life. He would have helped lay a healthy foundation for what the person thought about dentists. He would have explained to him why it was important for him to go regularly to the dentist, rather than waiting until the pain and discomfort forced him into making an appointment. And since this man would have likely had a different relationship with the dentist as an adult, he would have set a different example for his children, who also would have grown up with a better and healthier view of the dentist.

Believe me, who you choose as your dentist has a profound impact. Knowing how important good dental care is for your oral health, as well as for your emotional one, it just makes sense that not any dentist will do. Anyone can go to school to complete the necessary coursework to become a dentist. But not just anyone can be a great dentist. Along with the dental skills and knowledge, it takes people skills to also be a great dentist. You deserve a great dentist, and so does everyone in your family.

Making sure you have the best possible dentist for your family is an act of love. It helps to ensure their oral health needs will be met, which will be a great step toward helping to provide a safeguard for their emotional and overall health. It's a small act that has a big and effective outcome. There is simply too much at stake when it comes to oral health to just go to any dentist. It's imperative that you and your family have the best one, someone who will put your best interests in the forefront, and who understands people, as well as oral health.

Let's take a look at a few more reasons why not just any dentist will do. The internet has made it easy and efficient to get news from around the world. Decades ago, you only saw the news stories that made it to your local or national news, and it was a small fraction of what was really going on in the world. It was likely extremely rare that you ever heard the horror stories of what can happen when you don't have a great dentist. Today, that's all changed.

In today's news-filled world, it's easy to see what's going on in the dental world. You can quickly gain the latest research or read up on the best way to handle a minor discomfort. But you can also do a quick news search to see what the questionable dentists around the world are up to, because they make the headlines for those who are paying attention to them.

Do a couple of quick online searches and you are sure to find some of the dentist horror stories that have made the news in recent years. There are stories ranging from dentists being accused of harming and even torturing children, to those who did more work than they were supposed to, and some who did more harm than good. Some of the stories are enough to send shivers up your spine. I have no idea of the final outcome of the charges alleged in each of these news stories, but there's no doubt that there are some shady dentists out there.

Your mission is to find a dentist who isn't shady. You want to find a dentist who is the complete opposite and is considered excellent all the way around. Anything short of that and you will be selling you and your family short. The excellent dentists exist. It's just a matter of you opting for them to be your oral care partner. Once you do that, everything else will fall right into place.

Always remember that first impressions matter and can have a lifelong impact on how your children grow up to view dentists.

PROFESSIONALISM MATTERS

The dentist who is right for you and your family is one who is going to be professional in all areas of providing care. They will speak to you in a caring and open manner, maintain professionalism through-out every appointment, value your time, and be honest. Being able to trust your dentist is important so that you know the treatment being proposed is necessary and that you feel comfortable with all of the information you have received about it.

Along with professionalism, there are other factors that you need to consider when choosing a dentist. If at least most of these other areas don't fall into place with what you are looking for in a dental office, then obviously it is not a good fit. While you may have to compromise on something, you don't want to compromise on a lot, and you don't want to compromise on the bigger and more important issues. If you do compromise on the most important issues, you will spend time regretting it and likely soon be back to the drawing board to find another dentist.

Some of the other factors that demonstrate that not just any dentist will do for you and your family include:

- **Qualifications**. This should be a given, but the dentist's qualification are going to make a big difference. In order to have a great experience, you need a competent dentist. You need one who has the education, skills, and experience to provide you and your family with great care.

- **Location**. Where the dentist is located is going to make a difference to you. Everyone has a certain amount of time they are comfortable putting in to drive back and forth to the dentist. Beyond that, they will be close to the point of losing it, because they won't want to put the time in. Choosing a dentist who is in a geographic area you are comfortable with is going to help lay the foundation for a good relationship.

- **Expenses**. Most people have concerns regarding the cost of going to the dentist. Whether you have dental insurance or not, you want to make sure that the dentist you choose is going to be a good fit when it comes to costs. Make sure they work with your insurance, or if you are self-pay, find out if they accept such patients and what their terms are. We actually have our own dental plan, called the Advantage Plan, to help patients afford the care they need.

- **Emergency care**. Not just every dentist offers emergency care options. The last thing you want is to have a tooth knocked out, call your dentist, and get a recording or answering service that just tells you to go to the emergency room. A great dentist is going to want to be there to help you through those emergency situations.

- **Your comfort**. How comfortable you and your family members are when walking into a dentist office is important. When you walk into the right dentist's office you want to feel welcome, appreciated, and comfortable. You want to be comfortable not just with the dentist, but also with the hygienist and those who work in the office. Everyone should make you feel welcome and appreciated. Anything short of that just won't do.

- **Atmosphere**. Not just any dentist will do when it comes to the office atmosphere. Each year, there are complaints lodged to professional boards regarding particular dentist offices being dirty, for example. Once these boards receive the complaints they do go out and inspect the offices, but it's one more example of how just any dentist won't do. The dental office you go to should be impeccably clean, which helps to protect your health.

- **Ambience**. Face it, don't you want to go to a dental office that gives you a great vibe? Artwork, pictures, smiling faces, good looking uniforms, all the professional things that go along with quality service. It shows the office is successful, and they take their trade seriously.

Believe it or not, there are complaints filed each year regarding various dentist's personalities. The problem here is that while there are professional ethics that dentists should follow, there are no rules and regulations regarding one's personality. A governing board, for example, cannot tell a dentist that he or she needs a more pleasant attitude or a better personality. There are no guidelines about what your personality should be like, and it's not typically something that is taught in dental school.

The issue about the dentist's personality, however, is an important one. You need a dentist who has a personality that you are going to like. While it would be amazing to have someone who's personality is out of this world, you may not be able to find that, but you should be able to find someone who has a nice personality. You should have no problem finding someone who knows how to treat their patients well and show them that they appreciate having them as patients.

You want to know how I think patients should be treated? Well, in our offices we believe every patient should be treated like family. I want people to feel like they know us, to feel comfortable, and to feel a sense of belonging. If we set out to treat every patient like family, then we will be giving them the kind of treatment that we want to receive.

You deserve the same type of great treatment that a dentist would give his or her own family members, and nothing short of it.

If you were to ask ten people if they have any dental horror stories, there is a good chance that at least half of them will have something to share. Maybe it was a botched treatment, a missed issue, something they felt was done that didn't need to be, a dentist who made them feel ashamed, or one who made them afraid to see dentists regularly. The horror stories regarding dental care are vast. The best way to help prevent them from becoming stories that your family goes on to share is by doing everything within your power to find the best possible dentist for you and your family. Make the commitment to helping your family have the best dental and oral health experience. This will serve them well into the future, as well as helping to lay the foundation for future generations to also have a good dental experience.

CHAPTER 7

How to Know What Questions to Ask

Imagine getting a flyer in the mail from a new dentist office that has opened up three minutes from your home. The postcard looks nice and if offers an introductory special for new patients. It's enough to entice you to make an appointment, so you waste no time in getting it set up for the next week. Great, they got you into an appointment quickly, but does that mean you are all set and everything is going to go well?

Not so fast. A postcard that promotes a dentist may or may not be promoting the right dentist for you. And that goes for any other form of advertising or how the dentist office's information came your way to begin with. That person being advertised or referred to you by your best friend may be the best dentist in the world for you. Or maybe not. The only way you will know for sure is to do your own research.

> *Choosing the right dentist for your family means you must ask questions and get them all answered so that you can make an informed decision.*

Let's say the day of that appointment arrives that you were able to make so quickly and you go into their office. Upon walking in, you see the lobby is a bit dirty with cobwebs in the corner, outdated magazines on the tables, and a receptionist who doesn't acknowledge you. While you may be ready to withhold judgment so far, it could get worse. Maybe you go back into the exam room only to feel like you are being rushed around without anyone caring who you are, what your name is, or welcoming you as a new patient. The dentist walks in and it sends a chill up your spine because it feels like a cold front just moved in, again leaving you to wonder if you made the right decision.

The minute you start talking to the dentist about a cosmetic issue you want to get done, you have to go no further to realize you made a big mistake. The dentist gives you the vibe that they clearly are not an expert at cosmetic dentistry, and don't have the experience you want or need to handle your situation. You could run out of the office, but you fear tripping on the way out, causing a scene, or simply don't want to embarrass yourself like that. So you stick it out, only to feel you wasted your time on the way home, because you feel like it's back to the drawing board with searching for the right dentist for you and your family.

Without asking questions and getting everything you need answered, there is a good chance that you won't hit a home run and find the right dentist with limited effort. It would be fantastic if you could throw a dart at some names of dentists on the wall and whichever one it lands on was the right one. It would be equally fantastic if you could find that postcard from a dentist in your mailbox, make an appointment, and when you showed up everything felt great and you knew you were in the right place.

But that's just not how it usually happens. Finding the right dentist takes a little more work than that. One thing it absolutely takes is asking some questions. You can't possibly know if someone is the right dentist for you if you haven't asked some questions. And the questions that you ask are going to help make a world of difference in ensuring that you make the right choice.

Many people cringe at the thought of going through a series of questions with the dental office they are considering. They think it's going to take up a lot of time, be obtrusive, uncomfortable, and they would rather do a hundred other different things than spend their time doing that. I totally get that, but this is an area you cannot compromise on. Trust me when I say that asking the questions will actually save you a lot of time and discomfort in the long run.

Never feel bad about asking questions when you are choosing a dentist, or any doctor for that matter. This is one the most important aspects to being your best advocate. Patients must be their own best advocate, as it is the only way you will get the care that you are comfortable with and find a dentist that is a good fit for you.

MUST-HAVES FOR GREAT DENTAL CARE

Before we even get to the set of questions you will want to ask every dental office you are considering, there are some things that I consider must-haves in order for you to acquire great dental care. And you should not be settling for anything less than great dental care. Good or good enough care won't do, because there are great dentists out there who will do better than that. You deserve them, and they deserve you.

Here are the five must-haves that I believe must be present in order for you and your family to receive great dental care:

- **They care about you and your family**. The last thing you want is to just be another number or face that they don't remember, or where the staff is in a hurry to get you in and out of the office. You want to feel that they value and appreciate having your family there and that your treatment is important.

- **They are forthcoming in answering your questions to give you all of the information you need**. In order for you to make decisions and feel like an active part of the treatment, you need to know and understand what is going on. A great dentist never leaves you hanging with questions or uncertainty. You should always feel comfortable with what is going on, have an understanding of why things are being done the way they are, and feel as though all of your questions are answered. The questions you have should always be welcomed and addressed. If you have a dentist who seems too busy to answer you and you feel is too brief to actually provide you with the answers you are seeking, that could be a red flag.

- **They pay attention to your child, and not just you**. While parents may do a lot of the talking and decision making, it is often the kids who need treatment. It's important that the doctor make a connection with your child, helping them feel comfortable and heard. If they have concerns, they should feel comfortable expressing those concerns to the doctor, and the doctor should take the time to speak to them at their level, help them feel more comfortable, and show them they are valued as a patient.

- **They are open and honest with you about the treatment options**. You should be able to easily obtain information about such things as cleanings, examinations, fillings, braces, and much more. Along with the information and recommendations on these things, you should also be able to easily obtain information about what the treatments will cost and the types of finance options that are available to your family.

Remember, you are investing your time into taking your family to the dentist, and there is a lot that hangs in balance. It is crucial that you get great care to ensure that your investment pays off. When you have the right dentist by your side, it should feel like a partnership. You are both working together to help ensure that your child has their dental needs met in a satisfactory manner, with both of you doing your part.

When researching a dentist for your family, it is important to make sure that you verify they are board certified. When you have one in mind whom you are considering, set up a consultation with them. When you go into the office, pay attention to how you and your children are treated. From the greeting you get at the front desk through the appointment with the doctor, you should feel welcome and comfortable. Be sure to ask questions at that initial meeting so you know if this is the dentist you want to spend years seeing as your children grow up. It's also a good idea to see if there are reviews of the dentist's office online, and check with the Better Business Bureau to learn more about the reputation the office has.

WHAT QUESTIONS TO ASK

Asking questions where the dentist's office is located and if they are accepting new patients is always helpful, but your series of questions can't stop there. You need a lot more information to be able to evaluate each office you are considering. Asking the right questions will get you the answers you need to be able to evaluate, compare, and determine which dentist's office is the right one. Knowing the right questions to ask is going to help make it simple for you to narrow down the best dentist for you.

Here are some of the questions that you will want to ask every dentist's office that you interview for the position of your new family dentist:

1. **Is the dentist licensed?**

   You would think that if they are claiming to be a dentist that this is a given, that they must be licensed. Yet this is not always the case, and you can't be sure without inquiring to find out. All dentists need a license to practice, and to receive that they need to meet basic requirements, including an education requirement, a clinical requirement, and a written exam (requirements for dental licensing also vary by state). Additional training, degrees, and fellowships demonstrates expertise, extensive experience, advanced training, technological advancement in the field, and a commitment to the dental field. For instance, I am a fellow of the ICOI, the largest dental implant organization in the world.

2. **Is there a particular area that the dentist has extra experience in?**

This is an important question to ask so that you know what the dentist is spending most of their time on all week long. If they only see a few patients per year for cosmetic dentistry, then they will not have a lot of experience providing such treatments. Likewise, if you want a dentist who is child friendly, you want to ensure that the one you choose has many patients who are children, otherwise they won't have the experience you are looking for when it comes to treating children.

3. **What types of treatments are available at that dentist's office?**

There are many dentists who do not offer particular treatments, such as veneers, crowns, or extractions. It's always a good idea to know what the depth of service is going to be like. If the dentist doesn't do much beyond fillings, then you will be referred to someone else every time treatment is needed.

4. **Are there some real-life photos of people they have provided treatment to?**

Being able to see some before and after photos of some of the treatments they have provided to real-life people is huge. This will help you get an idea of what the dentist is capable of. Be sure you are not being shown stock photos. You don't want to see the work that a stranger did, you want to see what this particular dentist can do. Those who have the experience and are proud of the work they have done will be happy to show you before and after photos.

5. **Do they have testimonials from happy patients?**

Knowing that they have plenty of other satisfied patients can help bring you some comfort. Most dentists' offices that are worth their weight in gold can easily show you an array of testimonials. Be sure to read over the testimonials and see if the people were happy with their experience and what it is that they say they liked about the dentist and overall experience there. Don't feel like you have to stop at just reading the testimonials. There is nothing wrong with asking if they have a patient or two who you could speak with to inquire about their experience at the office. This will give you a chance to ask the patient questions that may help narrow down if the experience at that office will be good for you and your family.

6. **How many cases of a particular problem have they treated?**

If you want to know how many crowns a dentist has done, for example, you are better off asking how many cases they have completed. If you ask about cases, you will get a better idea of how many different patients the dentist has provided that treatment to.

7. **How many years has the dentist been providing services?**

While you want to know how long the person has been a dentist, you also should inquire about how long they have been providing specific treatments. If you know you need a porcelain veneer, you want to ask how many porcelain veneer cases they have completed and how long they have been providing the service.

8. **Does the dentist teach others and keep up on further education?**

Education is an important part of the dental field, but it should continue once dental school is over. Some dentists provide teaching and educational opportunities to others in the field. It's also important that they keep up on continuing education so they know what is new and are aware of the advancements in the industry. You can narrow the focus of the question by asking what type of continuing education did they have in the last year or so. Another great question is whether or not they have any written material. Do they lecture and offer seminars? All of these things show that the dentist is an authority in their field.

9. **Which laboratory do they use if things like veneers are crowns are needed?**

The quality of a porcelain veneer or crown is important and not something that should be ignored. There are plenty of labs that offer the services, while prices and quality vary widely. A quick online search of the lab they use can give you an idea if they use a quality one or not. Today there is a growing trend to use cheap dental labs in China and India. Many of these labs use substandard or even dangerous materials. You don't want your dentist cutting corners asking "How can we do this cheaper?" The quality and professionalism of the lab they use will have an impact on the quality of your treatment, should you need any of those services that call for lab work. You can always find it cheaper, but at what long-term cost? If your dental work needs replacing after a few years, did you really save any money?

10. **How much are treatments and what types of payment options are available?**

When you are asking this question, it helps if you already know on your end what your situation is. If you have dental insurance, you will want to know what it covers and how much you will be responsible for. Also, find out if it matters what dentist you go to, or if you have to choose from a particular list. If you have no dental insurance, inquire from the dental office what type of options they offer. Keep in mind that costs should not be your most important factor when choosing a dentist. It's great to know the information ahead of time, but it's never a good idea to choose a dentist based off of the price of treatments. When you are paying for a dental treatment, you are essentially paying for the dentist's expertise. You want a dentist who is well experienced and will provide the best, highest quality treatment. That's the main objective, not finding a dentist who has the lowest rates you can find.

11. **Does the dentist check for things like oral cancer and correct bite?**

> There are many important issues when it comes to oral care, and you need a dentist who will keep up on all of it. You want to ensure that the office does things like screen for oral cancer, checks for decay and gum disease, and will also ensure that you have a correct bite. Without having a correct bite, your teeth can break because of the stress, which makes it important that such things are considered.

These are eleven of the most important questions you will want to ask every dentist. By asking the right questions, you will get a deeper sense of what the dentist is capable of. These are things that may become a major issue later on if you don't know the answer to them from the start.

Most people don't take much effort in choosing the best dentist for them and their family. That's why they tend to go from dentist to dentist and end up with horror stories that they tell their friends. Problems that weren't treated correctly, issues that became worse, and more. Whether or not you like the treatment outcomes and your overall dental experience is going to come down to how much effort you put into finding the right dentist to begin with. You can avoid a lot of problems and headaches if you find the right dentist from the start. If you are happy with your teeth, you will be happier in general. So don't count the questions, make the questions count.

PHOTOS

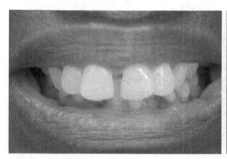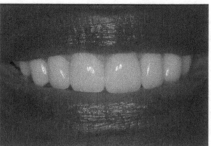

Diastema closure with eight porcelain veneers.

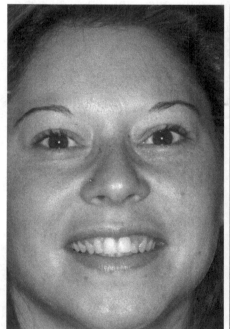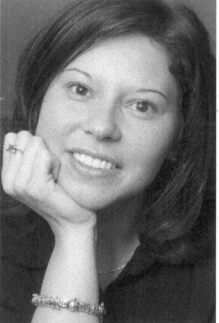

*Discolored, misaligned teeth and old crown
transformed with veneers and a new crown.*

PHOTOS

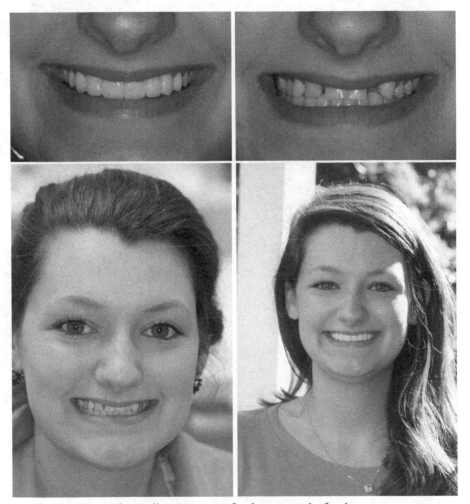

This girl actually came to me after being in ortho for three years.
We used veneers and a bridge to replace the front tooth.

PHOTOS

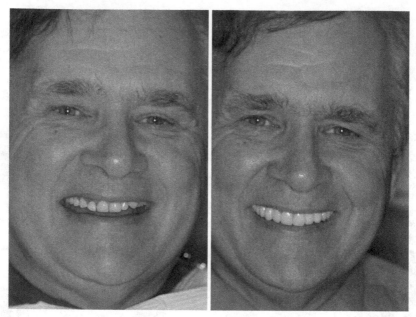

Extreme wear on all teeth and several fractured front teeth that were replaced with implants and crowns.

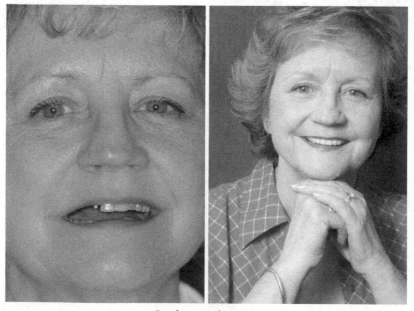

Implants and crowns.

PHOTOS

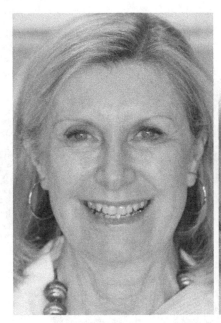
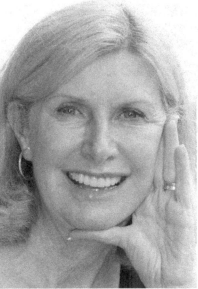

Instant orthodontics with eight veneers.

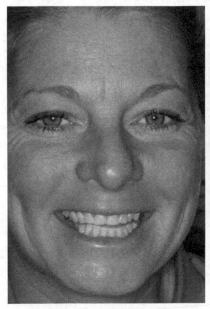
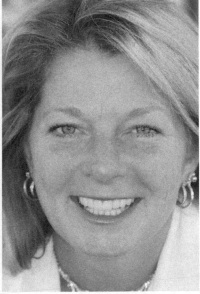

Extreme wear on teeth. A couple of implants were placed on the lower posterior.

PHOTOS

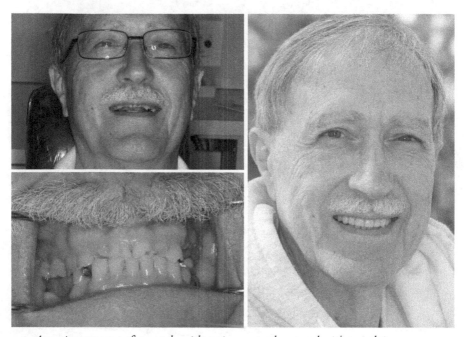

Amazing amount of stomach acid erosion on teeth restored with porcelain crowns.

PHOTOS

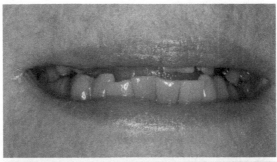

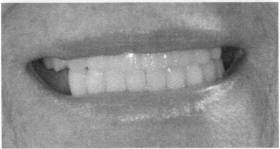

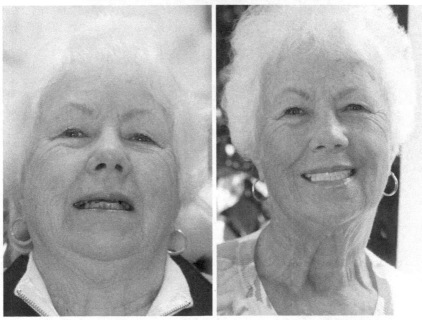

We restored this lady's mouth with wall-to-wall porcelain crowns and bridges. She was seventy-eight years old and wanted to have a great smile and improved chewing so she could be around for her grandkids longer.

CHAPTER 8

Why Not a Guarantee?

One of the questions you will want to ask any dentist you are considering is if they offer a guarantee. This is especially important if you are getting cosmetic dentistry, or will be having treatments done. If they raise an eyebrow and think that it's a strange question, ask why they do not offer a guarantee. In our offices, we have always offered one and always will.

Offering our patients a guarantee on the treatments that we provide is a way of letting them know we absolutely stand behind our work. We are committed to making sure that it's to their satisfaction and if there's a problem we won't leave them hanging. We will be there with them to help make it right until they are satisfied. Our relationship is a partnership, and we try to treat people like family. We wouldn't tell our family member that we are sorry they don't like the way it turned out and there's nothing that can be done. No, we would go to great lengths to help correct the problem, and it's the same thing we will do for every one of our patients.

The dentist you choose should be serious about standing behind their work.

But let's be honest, you may not get the response you want. You may be told there are no guarantees. In fact, you may be made to feel like it's out of the question to ask such a question. Don't be surprised if this happens to you at more than one dental office, but know that there are dentists out there who stand by their work and will offer a guarantee.

Health care is notorious for no guarantees. Surgeons have a dark-humor insiders' joke: Dead patients can't sue. If you've seen reality TV shows about plastic surgery, like the popular one called *BOTCHED*, you know things can go horribly wrong. Guarantees are controversial in all kinds of health care including orthodontics. Many doctors are upset by the very idea. One huffed-and-puffed at me, "What do you think you're doing with this guarantee nonsense? We aren't operating Midas Muffler® shops, installing mufflers and guaranteeing them for five thousand miles. We are doctors, dammit." His doctor-ego was mightily offended. But I doubt you will be, with the challenge of deciding who should be your family's trusted dentist. So, yes, I think there should be a guarantee. In fact, guarantees.

Here are some of the guarantees that I offer. The dentist you choose should be making similar guarantees on the work that they do, whether it's on porcelain veneers, crowns, or root canals. They should stand by their work and provide you with the treatment that you deserve.

1. If you aren't satisfied with your treatment, new smile outcome or patient/parent experience, we will remake your veneers.

2. You have a safety in numbers guarantee. Top dentists nationwide treat more than one million patients successfully with the diagnostic and prescriptive methods, state of the art technology, and techniques we use. Here, in my Irmo office, we treat many patients per year. Our reputation is stellar. What patients and their parents say in their own words is revealing, and we offer an array of testimonials for people to see.

3. You have my guarantee that every dentist and dental assistant at my office has been not only academically educated, but also thoroughly trained in my treatment method—exactly how I diagnose needs, plan best treatment, customize treatment to each patient, and manage for best results from day-one through after-care. There is nobody learning on the job with you or your child. Ever. All patient care is supervised and reviewed by me. We also invest in frequent state-of-the-art clinical continuing education for our team, exceeding all state licensing requirements above and beyond.

4. You also have my guarantee of exceptional courtesy and customer service. I invest in training for the entire team by celebrated organizations like the Disney Institute and Ritz-Carlton. And yes, you are my patient, but we can be honest about this—my practice is not just a health care provider, it is a business. As such, it has, in my opinion, one set of responsibilities to you as the parent of a patient

and to the patient, including telling the whole truth and nothing but the truth, prescribing in the patient's best interest, and delivering the best possible treatment and outcomes. As well as responsibilities to you as a customer, including access, convenience, responsiveness, and red carpet service. My staff can tell you: I flip out if we drop the ball. You are even given my personal, executive assistant's direct cellphone number. She will either step in to fix whatever ails for you, or she can—and will—get to me pronto, regardless of where I may be. I have zero tolerance for legitimately dissatisfied customers.

These guarantees are included in your treatment program fee. As a dentist, I know how important it is to people that they trust what they are signing up for. They need to know that the time and money invested in their treatment will not be wasted. At my office, we go above and beyond when it comes to providing excellent patient services and care, and we stand behind everything we do. We believe in doing things to the best of our ability, which helps keep our patients happy, which makes us happy in return.

The dentist you choose should offer some type of guarantee on the treatments that you will be having done. If they offer a guarantee, find out what it includes. Some may call it a warranty on the work as well, but again you want to know exactly what that means. There are some dentists who may offer a guarantee on their work, but it may also come with the stipulation that you remain a patient of theirs for five years after receiving the treatment.

You want to be well aware of the terms and conditions of the guarantee or warranty that they are offering, so you can see if it's legitimate, or something they are trying to pass as being an honest backing of their work. Your dentist should want you to feel confident with the decision to have your treatment done at their office. If they provide high-quality care, then they should also offer a guarantee.

THE TYPE OF GUARANTEE

Typically, if the dentist is going to back the work they do, they will offer it on the services that they provide. These include such treatments as dental fillings, implants, crowns, and bridges. When people get braces in my office, I want to make absolutely certain that they are happy with the outcome, and I guarantee to help them get there.

What people are generally protected against when it comes to dentist guarantees are breakage, loosening, detachment, or decay that may happen under the restoration. This is important to have, because the last thing you want is to put out $3,000 on two crowns only to have one break or fall off six months later. Without the dentist guaranteeing the work that they have done, where will that leave you? It would leave you shelling out more money to get it fixed. What if it doesn't last this time?

You simply can't put out the kind of money that it costs for dental treatments and not get some kind of guarantee that the dentist will be there to help make things right if something goes wrong. The average cost of a dental bridge is around $1,500 per tooth, and porcelain crowns can cost up to $2,000 per tooth. That's a significant investment you are making, and you need some kind of guarantee that it's going to do what you are paying for.

You wouldn't go purchase a large screen television without the ability to have it replaced or repaired if three months later it stopped working. We don't spend that kind of money without trusting that we are going to be able to use it for a while and it's going to do what it's intended to do. The same concept holds true with dental work.

If you pay for dental work, you should be able to trust that it's going to hold up for the amount of time that the dentist advised it would. As long as you maintain your part of the bargain—wear nightguards, come in for regular cleanings, and even refer your friends—we will work together like partners to help you too.

A guarantee from the dentist doesn't mean you can go be reckless with the tooth and run back and get it fixed. Dentists are going to provide you with instructions on how to care for the treatment that you had done, and in order to be eligible for the guarantee, you are going to have live up to your end of the deal by following their instructions and taking care of the teeth that had the treatments.

While you want the guarantee on the work, you also need to be aware that routine lifespan won't be covered. And that's a fair thing, and as it should be. You wouldn't expect to get a crown, for example, and assume that it will last you the rest of your life and if it doesn't, then the dentist will fix it and have you on your way. The lifespan of a crown greatly varies. Some people may find that they last ten years, but others may have one that lasts thirty years. Be sure to ask the dentist how long you can expect the work that is being performed to last. Having an honest assessment will let you know what to expect to get out of it in terms of lifespan.

Any dentist's office that believes in the quality of what they are doing will offer a guarantee of some kind. Knowing what that guarantee is and what is included is the best way to know how confident they are in their work and what you can expect if something were to go wrong. When you invest in your teeth, you want to feel confident and comfortable that you will get what you are paying for, and that it will be of high quality.

WHAT INVALIDATES A GUARANTEE

If the dentist offers a guarantee, you want to know what will invalidate it as well. This information should be in written form so that you can keep the information and refer back to it. Not having it from the start opens the door to interpretation later that could cause issues. It's like playing a game without both sides being aware of what the rules are. Everyone needs to go into this knowing what the rules are. So find out what the guarantee is, and what types of things would invalidate it.

Of course, this will vary for every dentist who offers a guarantee, but it gives you an idea of what to watch for and inquire about. They include such things as:

- **Not returning to the dentist for a routine check-up at least once a year during the period for which they guaranteed the work that was done**. Most dentists who offer a guarantee will want you to keep up your end of good oral hygiene practices, which includes keep up with your preventive checkups.

- **Not keeping up with your oral hygiene practices**. Let's say that you go get some work done and then you decide you no longer feel like doing the work to keep up on brushing your teeth. I know it seems crazy, but trust me, there are people who fall into lazy habits and they stop brushing or they get haphazard, only brushing periodically.

- **Not following the instructions that the dentist provided for caring for the work that was done**. If there is something specific that you were informed needed to be done to care for the work, then you will have to hold up your end of the bargain by following through with doing those tasks. The dentist will be clear about providing you with that information before the work is done, so that you are not blindsided with it later on.

- **Accidents that may cause harm to the work that was done**. What this means is that your husband doesn't get a bridge put in and then a couple of months later while playing on the men's basketball team he takes an elbow to the mouth while guarding a game-winning shot. If that elbow to the mouth breaks or damages the bridge, then it won't fall under the guarantee for the dentist to fix it free of charge.

- **Illnesses that you may have or get that lead to damage in your teeth, gums or bones in the mouth**. For example, if you have diabetes, epilepsy, or you undergo chemotherapy, it may have a negative effect on your dental condition. This is something that is beyond the scope of the work that the dentist provided, so it wouldn't be covered under the guarantee in most cases.

The guarantee that you get from a dentist isn't a free-for-all so that you can treat your teeth any old way you want and then head back into the office expecting them to repair it under the guise of their guarantee. You want a guarantee that will cover the work that they did and their craftsmanship. You want the work to be of high quality, so that when you walk out the door you are confident that the bridge is going to hold up, or the fillings you just had put in are not going to fall apart or fall out a week later.

A dentist who is confident with the work they do will offer some type of guarantee on it. They will stand behind their treatments and they will be forthcoming in letting you know ahead of time what to expect, how to care for the work they have done, what the guarantee covers, and what your end of the arrangement is. This is fair, and this is a sign of a good dentist.

The amount of time that a dentist will guarantee the work for that they are doing also varies, but it's reasonable for you to find a five-year guarantee on a bridge or inlay, a three-year guarantee on ceramic veneers, three to four years on a combination treatment of a crown and bridge, a year on a full set of dentures, and a year on composite fillings. This gives you something to look for and ask about, so that you have the peace of mind for that time frame that the work they are providing will hold up on its own, without outside forces (such as accidents or neglect) causing problems.

PREVENTION SOLUTIONS

A dentist's office that provides a guarantee is one that shows they believe in a long-term commitment to your dental health. They will also be forthcoming with the information on how to care for your teeth between dental visits, so that you can extend the life of any of your dental work, and you can help to have better oral hygiene and health all the way around. Much of the information they provide is geared toward prevention, as it should be.

Prevention is the best way to take care of our health, and the same goes for our oral health. When we take steps to take care of our teeth, gums, and overall oral health, we will be in a better position to help avoid needing treatments in the first place. Preventative dentistry, which is caring for the teeth in order to help keep them healthy and prevent problems, should be high on everyone's priority list.

Many people focus on children when it comes to dental problems, but adults get plenty of them as well. It's imperative to maintain good dental hygiene practices all throughout your life, from childhood into old age. By keeping up on your regular dental visits, you will be doing a world of good in helping to care for your overall dental health, as well as your general health.

If the dentists you interview for the position do not offer a guarantee, ask them why not. As someone who will be investing time and money, you deserve a guarantee that will help ensure you are receiving great treatment, and that the dentist stands behind the work that they do. Finding a dentist who guarantees the work that they do should not be difficult, but it is something that will help you sort through candidates in order to narrow down the list to the better ones.

In my office we offer guarantees, because we stand by our work and we are committed to the patients' long-term oral health. Your dentist should feel the same way, or it may not be the right dentist for you and your family. You deserve a guarantee, and there is a great dentist out there who is ready to offer you one.

CHAPTER 9

How to Tackle the Ugly Matter of Money

You know it's coming and I know it's coming. We can't possibly have a discussion about dental work without having the discussion about how it's going to be paid for. Like any other type of medical or health services, taking care of your teeth and oral health comes at a price. Granted, it's a smart investment and well worth making, but you still need the info how to get the bill paid for when the time comes. Relax. This is an area where most people tend to focus on too much, and worry far more than they need to.

Yes, whatever work you have done going to the dentist is going to come with a bill, but that's to be expected. Depending on what services and treatments are being done, it could range from $100 for a cleaning and exam to thousands of dollars for restorative dentistry.

Still, there's no need to panic at this point. You will be able to pay your dental tab without breaking the bank.

Whether or not you have dental insurance, you may still be paying for some of your bill out of pocket. Dental insurance doesn't usually pick up the tab for everything, so you should expect that you will be paying a portion. What portion becomes your responsibility will be determined by what procedures you have done. Some things cost more than others. For example, if you are merely going for a cleaning and exam, that's not something costly and you won't need to take loans for it. But if you need several crowns or your child needs braces, that's going to be in the thousands and there's a good chance that you will need some payment options.

The good news is that payment options are usually available. Just about every dentist and I've ever spoken to does offer some sort of payment options. They expect that patients will need the information, and so they usually have it ready for you when you need it. They have looked into the options that are available, have compiled the info, and can offer you what they know to be the best routes for you to consider. Of course, you can go beyond that and do some research on your own, too, but what they are offering is a good starting place.

The first thing you will want to do is find out the specifics of your insurance policy, because that is going to have a lot to do with how much you end up paying out of pocket. Some insurance plans may pay for just about everything, while others may split the cost with you, or only pay a small portion. There are many different types of dental insurance plans out there, with each of them offering a variety of plans. One way that many people help pay for their dental bills is through using their benefits known as "flex spending," where an account with their job can be used to pay for dental bills through pre-tax dollars.

AVOIDING FLEX SPENDING HEADACHES

Some people find that flex spending arrangements are a headache and they may even try to avoid them, at times avoiding the dental work all together or paying for it another way. The good news is that there are ways that you can help to eliminate the flex spending headaches. It all comes down to knowing what to do to make it easier and avoid the stress that comes with such accounts if you don't plan ahead.

There are three main solutions you can take to get the most out of your employer's flex plan so that the amount out of your pocket is reduced to a more manageable figure. Here are the three solutions you can start taking action with today:

1. **Sign up early**. Preparation is key to success in any endeavor. So make the most of your flex plan. Set aside your flex spending dollars now. Many employers set higher limits than you think on the amount of flex spending dollars you can contribute each year, tax free, from your salary to pay for health care expenses, such as dental care. Case in point: Many employers allow $2,500, or even $5,000 of pre-tax earnings to be set aside for your flex plan. Are you getting all of that money you can to pay for your family's dental care? You may not be. If you fail to sign up early, it could cost you more out-of-pocket for dental expenses, especially if your plan is not set up and ready before the treatment begins. If you have a new plan, work with your plan administrator to sign up early for next year in order to help maximize your savings.

2. **Make sure your employer is aware of any family status change**. Employers all have their own sign-up deadlines for flex plans, but typically at the beginning of the year,

your employer asks you how much money you want to contribute to your flex plan for the year. The problem with making annual decisions about your healthcare coverage is that you only have the opportunity to enroll, unless you have a qualified "family status change." What exactly is a family status change? They are things like marriage, divorce, births, and a loss of a spouse's insurance coverage. Each of these status changes is a qualified reason to change your plan, and possibly add more coverage for dental care, yet most people are not aware of it.

3. **Choose wisely**. Finally, give some thought to calculating how much money to contribute to your flex plan at work this year. If you are considering some cosmetic dentistry or orthodontic treatments, visit your doctor's offices for the initial consultation. Their office can help you plan exactly how much money you should contribute to help reduce your out-of-pocket expenses when it's time to pay for, and receive, the procedure you are inquiring about.

Here's something you may not know about your flex plan: If you put in more money than you need, by law, you lose the money. You have three months after the end of the calendar year to submit claims for eligible expenses from the previous calendar year. Any money left in your account after this three-month period is lost.

THE SCOOP ON INSURANCE

I can tell you that today there are as many different types of insurance as there are patients. And every one of them tends to be a bit different, all offering something unique, and paying for different things in varying amounts. I can't possibly speak to your specific and unique insurance policy without seeing it first, but I can say that in my experience, most dental insurance is going to cover some of your expenses beyond a yearly exam and cleaning. What amount they cover is going to be the part that varies, and will be information you will want to know ahead of time.

If you don't have dental benefits, or you would like to make a switch to find a better plan, you are in luck. There are many dental insurance plans and they are often quite affordable. Remember, that the dental insurance you have, especially if it is through your employment, chosen by your employer, who determines the amount of benefits you would receive! Some of the different types of dental insurance plans that are offered include:

- **Table or schedule of allowance plans**. These plans have a pre-determined list of treatments and what they will pay for each of them. The information stays consistent regardless of where you go for treatment. Whatever the difference is between what they will pay for the treatment and what the dentist bills you for would be your responsibility to pay. Unless you have a secondary insurance plan to pick up that extra, you will be paying that out-of-pocket.

- **Direct reimbursement programs**. This type of dental insurance plan comes with a pre-determined amount or percentage that the company will pay toward your dental care. With this type of plan, you can usually go to the dentist of your choice. They may say, for example, that they will pay 50 percent of the bill on all of your crowns, veneers, or bridges. If this is the case, you may want to work with the dentist to get the best possible rate, since it will save you from paying more out of your own pocket.

- **UCR plans**, which stands for "usual, customary, and reasonable," which is a plan that will pay a usual, customary, or reasonable fee to the dentist for the services rendered. The patient can usually choose which dentist they want to go to as well. With this type of plan, the insurance company has a payment agreement with the dentist's office.

Again, dental insurance plans vary, so you have to choose the one that is going to be the best for your family. Know what it covers and what is expected of you. Find out if it requires you go to a specific dentist's office, or if you can choose your own dentist (most allow you to go to any dentist you want). You want to be able to choose your own dentist, because you can't possibly find the best dentist for your family by letting someone else make that decision for you (especially allowing an insurance company to make that decision for you).

Never let money keep you from having good oral health. It's too important to overlook and skip it.

Some plans will require that you make a co-payment, and others may state that you have to get pre-approval to get treatment, such as cosmetic dentistry, done. These things will all vary by company, but in order to get the most out of your health insurance plan you have to know what the details of it are. Know what it covers, what you will be responsible for, and what your responsibility as a patient will be, so that you can make the insurance work to your benefit.

Most insurance plans will come with an annual benefit limitation. This means that they are only willing to spend a particular amount of money per year on your treatment. This is fine, but you need to know what that amount is. Knowing what it is will help keep you from exceeding it, and will also help you to get the most out of it. You can be more effective at planning your dental care treatment when you know what your yearly benefit limitation is.

Some of the questions you will want to keep in mind when choosing a dental insurance plan include:

- **Will you be able to choose your own dentist**? You are reading this book because you want to know how to choose the best possible dentist for you and your family. So, if you are not the one choosing the dentist office you go to, then that should be a red flag. Unless the dentist you go to is on that list, think twice about choosing that dental insurance plan.

- **Will it be your dentist or your insurance company that is deciding on whether or not you have treatment done**? You want it to be your dentist who makes the decisions, not the insurance company. If you have the right dentist for you, then you can trust that the treatment they are recommending is something that is necessary.

- **What does the insurance plan cover**? Does it cover emergency services, preventative measures, and diagnostic appointments?

- **How much of the dental bill will you be responsible for**? What percentage of the treatment do they cover?

- **What type of benefit limitations are there**, and are there any treatments that are excluded?

- **What is their policy if your dentist refers you to a specialist**?

When choosing the right dental insurance plan, you want to consider every member of your family and what their possible treatment recommendations may be. If you know that someone in the family may need braces, crowns, or fillings, keep that in mind as you check out the various plans and see what they cover.

The Internet has made it easier for people to shop around for dental insurance plans. Within minutes, you can compare rates and plans, so that you can find the best one for you. Finding the right insurance plan for you and your family goes hand-in-hand with choosing the right dentist.

SELF-PAY OPTIONS

There are many people who have no dental insurance at all, and there are many others who have insurance but can't afford to pay cash for their out-of-pocket expenses for their treatments. This is more common than you may realize, so if you fall into this category you shouldn't feel down about it, and you also shouldn't avoid seeing the dentist. You need the treatments every bit as much as others with insurance, so don't let the lack of insurance keep you from getting it.

There are always options for those who are considered self-pay patients. For those who are self-pay and have the cash to pay the bill outright, then that's their plan and they usually need nothing in addition to it. But for the many who don't have a couple of extra thousand laying around to pay the tab for their dental work, they may need to speak to the dentist's office about payment options.

Most dental offices are well prepared to provide you with information and options regarding ways to pay. Some may offer to let you make the payments directly to the dentist's office and spread the payments out of a specified amount of time. Others may like their patients to go with a small loan service, such as Care Credit. With Care Credit, you can get a small loan to pay for the treatment you need, and then make the payments back monthly, for the agreed-upon length of the loan. This gives people a year or two, or the amount of time agreed upon, to pay for the treatment they need.

With something like Care Credit, it typically covers a wide range of treatments, including periodontal scaling, sealants, teeth cleaning, dental implants, root canals, ceramic crowns, braces and retainers, veneers, tooth repair, and more. If there is a treatment that you need or want, there is a good chance that Care Credit can offer the financing to help make it happen. They allot for an amount that typically covers a good portion of the treatment, if not all of it. For a porcelain veneer, for example, they will loan up to $2,500 per tooth, and for composite veneers they will loan up to $1,500 per tooth.

There are additional loan options available, so if there is a treatment you need to take one out for, be sure to shop around and weigh your options to get the best rate. Find something you are comfortable with, so that you can afford the monthly payment and can still get the treatment you need.

It's also a good idea to speak with the dentist's office if you are a self-pay patient. They will want to work with you to help point you in the right direction to be able to find financing and payment options. We offer our own Advantage Plan to patients who have minimal or no dental insurance, to help them cover their costs.

Additional options you will want to consider, should you need to, include your own personal financing options. Check with your credit card companies, credit union, and other such places to see what type of loan options are available. Once you have all the information available to you, then you can choose the best route to take.

ADDITIONAL THOUGHTS

Often times, people will put off dental work that they need, because they don't want to spend the money. They tend to think that by avoiding the work they are saving money, or at least not spending any. But that isn't always the case. Most of the time when it comes to dental work that is needed, the longer you put it off, the more expensive it will be to treat when you finally do go in to have it done. In the dental world, things tend to get worse and it leads to bigger, more serious problems that will be more costly to address. It's always a good idea to avoid putting dental work off. Get it done when you first need it, so that it doesn't get worse and end up costing you more down the road.

Knowing what your payment options are and what's available to you, work with the dentist to space out your treatment if you need to. If you need to space the treatment out throughout the year, it will help to spread the payments out, and make it easier for many people. The options are always there, it's just a matter of discussing it with the dentist to see what can be done.

Is going to the dentist expensive? No, it's not going to the dentist that is expensive. Remember, there is a lot that is at stake when it comes to your oral health. It impacts many areas of your life, including your overall health, emotional well-being and your overall quality of life. When you add up all that can be harmed by not going to the dentist to have treatments done, it's easy to see that the costly option is to avoid the dentist all together.

Whether you have dental insurance, need loans to pay for your services, or will be paying cash, there are options for everyone. The key is to know what you have available to you, what everyone in your family needs in terms of treatment, and to evaluate your options. When you let the dentist know what you are thinking and that you need to know the options, you will find that it's easier to find a plan that meets your needs. And when you look in the mirror and see that great smile, you will be glad you stuck with it to find the right payment plan for you and your family.

CHAPTER 10

Is Sedation Dentistry
a Good Idea?

Every year around the country, there are millions of people who have such fear of going to the dentist that they just skip it. Yes, the fear of all the what-ifs and what could happen consumes them to the point that they literally don't ever go to the dentist. This is the case whether they are in pain or they simply need a routine cleaning. They continue to avoid the dentist, allowing the fear and anxiety to rule supreme.

Meanwhile, what happens is that their teeth end up having more and more problems. If you are someone who avoids going to the dentist out of fear, there is a good chance that you will end up having more oral health problems. And as we know from previous chapters, poor oral health can increase chances of poor overall health. So what is it exactly that creates this heightened sense of fear regarding to the dentist, and what can be done about it? That's the important question for everyone who has experienced this, or who has a loved one who needs information, so that they can overcome this problem.

We must remember that our overall health is tied to our oral health. The more we understand the problem of fear and anxiety that people have for going to the dentist, the more we will be able to tackle the problem. Without addressing it, those who have the fear will likely suffer from poor oral health. Plus, our smile says a lot about us. What happens if you always avoid the dentist? What can a smile that never goes the dentist say about the person? There is a good chance they will not have the smile and teeth they wish they did, and it will hold them back from a lot of things. They will tend to be less confident and may avoid many social situations as a result.

WHY PEOPLE HAVE DENTAL FEAR AND ANXIETY

For the millions of people who have an extreme fear of going to the dentist, the reasons may vary as much as the people themselves. There is no one definitive reason why someone has such anxiety about going to the dentist that it prompts them to literally feel sick and avoid it at all costs. Some people have such anxiety about the dentist because of childhood experiences gone wrong. They may have gone to a dentist who scared or hurt them, and it created a lasting image that made them fearful to ever go back to another one.

This is one of the reasons why it is so important to find the right dentist for your family. We all know how important first impressions are, and you don't get a second chance to make a first impression. If a child goes to a dentist and it's not a good experience for them, then there is a good chance that will set the tone for future visits. They will become fearful and try to avoid going to the dentist. There are some people who are able to overcome this, often because their next experience with a different dentist was able to change their image and mindset, but that's not always the case. More often than not, if a child has a poor dental experience while they are young, they will grow up to think poorly about going to the dentist as an adult. If the experience was really bad, they may end up being one of the millions of people who at the mere thought of going for an appointment end up with anxiety, feeling sick, or becoming so upset that they literally can't go to the appointment.

Other factors that can contribute to people being overly fearful of going to the dentist include hearing other people's horror stories, or watching videos and movies. There are videos and movies that put dental horror stories out there into the mainstream, and it can give people a lot of reason to be afraid to step foot into an dentist office. Still others may have a gag reflex that makes them afraid to go to the dentist. When they have their mouth open and work is being done, they may continuously and unintentionally gag. They fear they are going to choke, and this can cause some serious anxiety about being in the dental chair.

It's estimated that up to 45 million people in the US have fear and anxiety to the point that they avoid seeing the dentist.

Some people may suffer from anxiety about going to the dentist and some may have a phobia. We all experience some anxiety at times, as it can be a normal part of life. Some anxiety is even good for us, because it helps make us more alert and cautious in life and can help protect us. Those with anxiety about going to the dentist may feel nervous about their appointment, but many will still go to it. Those with a phobia regarding going to the dentist will avoid it at all costs. They believe they will be in real danger if they attend the appointment. It's an irrational fear about going when there is no real danger.

Those with a phobia about going to the dentist may experience panic, fear, rapid heartbeat, shortness of breath, trembling, and an intense desire to get away. Their fight or flight instincts have told them there is danger and they need to get the out of dodge in order to protect themselves.

Other people who may consider using sedation dentistry are those who have difficulty sitting still. There are many people who have hyperactivity disorders and it is very difficult for them to sit still, especially for the amount of time that it may take to complete a procedure. Those who also have a low threshold for pain or who have very sensitive teeth may consider sedation dentistry. Both of these conditions could add to the fear and anxiety they experience at the dentist. Additionally, if there is someone who has a lot of work that needs to be done, they may be able to get more of it done at once by using sedation dentistry techniques. This could help cut down on the number of appointments that they need to go to in order to get all the work completed.

Whether you or someone in your family have an intense anxiety or phobia about going to the dentist, it's important to find ways to overcome that. Your oral health is too important to ignore because of an irrational fear. The good news is that with today's technology there are ways to help people move past their fears so that they can go to the dentist and still have great oral health.

DENTAL SEDATION

An option that many people consider when it comes to being fearful of going to the dentist is sedation dentistry. It has become popular in recent years with both children and adults. Many people see it as the answer to help those who fear the dentist to be able to get past the fear and get the dental treatment that they need. But is it a good idea to opt for sedation dentistry? You can only answer that question when you know what it is, what all it involves, and what the alternatives may be.

Sedation dentistry, sometimes referred to as "snooze" dentistry, is the use of medication in order to help patients relax and move past their fear and anxiety. It's been around for a long time, but in recent years there have been many dentists who are promoting it, and many patients who are jumping at the chance to check it out and see if it helps them be able to get the appointment over without all the fear and anxiety. The medications that are used give the patient the ability to overcome the fear, without them having to try to do it all on their own. Left to try and overcome the fear on their own, many would never be able to do it.

There are various types of sedation dentistry, so it is important if you are considering it to speak with the dentist about which ones their office offers. These include:

- **Oral sedation**—This involves the patient taking a pill, usually about an hour before their appointment, then having someone else drive them to the dentist's office. Once there, they will be taken into care of the dental staff, who will see them through the appointment. The sedation keeps the person awake, but helps them to relax and be more comfortable throughout the appointment.

Following the appointment, the patient would need to be driven home by someone else.

- **Nitrous oxide**—Otherwise known as "laughing gas," this type of sedation is administered by placing a mask over the nose. The person would breathe in the nitrous oxide, which would help them to relax and have a more comfortable experience through the appointment. If the inhaled sedation is minimal, the person may be able to drive themselves home.

- **IV sedation**—This type of sedation administers the drug through an IV, so it works faster. Usually this is administered by an oral surgeon. The surgeon can also adjust the amount that is being administered to the patient as the appointment goes along.

- **General anesthetic**—With this practice, the patient is not awake during the procedure. This is rarely used, except on special cases in the OR (Operating Room).

Sedation can range, being minimal, moderate, or deep, as well as the person being completely unconscious while under general anesthesia. Depending on the one that the person opts for, this will determine whether or not they are able to drive home on their own or if they need someone to do the driving for them. In addition to the sedation, a local anesthesia is still used in the mouth where the work will be performed. The local anesthesia is to keep the patient from feeling pain when the work is being done.

When considering whether or not sedation dentistry is a good idea for you, it's always wise to weigh the pros and cons and consider the alternative options. It can be a great way to help those who have anxiety and phobias be able to get the dental work done that they need, and to help them keep up with good oral health. The medications used for oral sedation are considered safe, and they have been found to be very effective in helping people to relax so they can get their dental work done.

There are a few downsides to using some of the particular medications, which include that they can take a while to be effective. This means that, depending on when it was taken, it may not yet be effective when the appointment time comes. Also, it could be challenging to determine the best dosage that someone should take in order to achieve the desired results, and they can't usually be adjusted once the procedure is underway. There is also a limit to how much can be taken, so if someone needs more than what is allowed they may not be able to get the effect that is needed in order to have a comfortable appointment. Also, some of the medications can create a type of hangover, which will leave people feeling a little spaced out, and it can last for even a couple of days.

When it comes to children, there are dentists who offer sedation dentistry. The American Academy of Pediatrics recommends that parents have thorough knowledge about the sedation and what to expect, so that they can help their child through the process to help ensure a successful outcome. Their recommendation is that parents can help children to prepare for the appointment, and know what to do during and after the appointment. They offer detailed guidelines for parents on their website. Sedation use on children is controversial, as there are some people on both sides of the issue, with some for and against the use of it. If you are considering using sedation dentistry on your child, speak with the dentist, as well as your pediatrician, to get opinions and recommendations. The costs of sedation dentistry vary, depending on the type you will be getting. They range from around $75-90 for nitrous oxide, to $300-400 for oral sedation, and around $600 for IV sedation.

Not every dentist's office will offer these types of sedation dentistry. Some of the types of sedation require training and that emergency supplies be on hand. Most states require that the dentist have a license to offer sedation dentistry, so you will need to inquire about what types the particular dentist you are considering going to offers. If you are going to have sedation dentistry done, you want to make sure you are with a dentist who is well experienced and qualified in providing it. The dental board in your state determines the license required to administer sedation dentistry. You have the ability to inquire with them about what is required in your state.

If you have health conditions, such as diabetes, cardiac conditions, hypertension, or other serious issues, be sure to speak with your physician about sedation dentistry if you are considering having it done. It's always a good idea to get their approval to go ahead with it, as they will be more familiar with your overall health and know if you are a good candidate for it or not.

WHAT THE SCIENCE SAYS AND THE ALTERNATIVES

Over the years, there have been studies that focused on sedation dentistry. This is always a good thing, because it provides us with a little something to back up the ideas behind the practice. In the April 2016 issue of the journal *Dental Clinics of North America*, they report that orally administered sedation is useful for treatment of anxious adults and pediatrics patients. They state that it is a cost-effective and effective service that is widely available, and enables the dentist to provide care to millions who would otherwise have their dental needs unmet.

The Centers for Disease Control and Prevention reports that almost 19 percent of children and nearly 32 percent of adults have untreated dental issues; meaning millions of children and adults are walking around with cavities in their mouth left untreated. If some of those are due to fear and anxiety over going to the dentist, and millions of them would have to be, then sedation dentistry is going to provide a good option for them to consider. There can be some terrible consequences to not getting dental work done, which makes sedation dentistry a solution that should be considered for those who would otherwise go without getting the work done at all.

For those who have concerns about sedation dentistry and want to explore alternatives to overcoming the anxiety or phobia, there are options. One of the most important things you can do for your family in order to overcome dental anxiety is to find the right dentist to begin with. The right dentist will be the first step in helping to put the person at ease and make them feel comfortable. They will be understanding of their fears and anxiety and help to alleviate it, as well as offer options for overcoming it, including ones that don't involve sedation dentistry.

It's important for those who have anxiety and phobias about the dentist to recognize it, and to talk about it. When they discuss it with their dentist, they may discover ways to work through it, so that the dental work can still be done. The patient can also work through it by starting with short and easy appointments, and work their way up to ones that require more work. This way they will feel more comfortable with each visit. They may also be more comfortable if they can bring a trusted person with them to the appointment, so that it helps to calm them down and feel safer.

Additionally, it's a good idea for the person to learn distraction methods, so that they are not focused on thinking about the dentist's appointment, and to learn relaxation techniques. Using something like a television show or headphones will help to distract the patient while work is being performed. Relaxation techniques, which can be useful in many situations in life, can help to immediately relax people. They include focusing on breathing, where your attention is turned to just focusing on the breath. This is a type of mediation that helps to calm you down. Also, using a visualization technique can be helpful, as the person keeps their mind focused on something positive that they enjoy, such relaxing at the beach.

Those who have a serious phobia regarding going to the dentist may benefit from speaking with a psychologist. They can help the person to work through the problem and possibly move past it so that they can become more comfortable going to the dentist.

MAKING THE CALL

So, we are brought back to our original question: Is sedation dentistry a good idea? The bottom line regarding that is yes, for many people it is a good idea. There are some people who would otherwise not get the dental treatment they need without having the option of using sedation dentistry. For that reason alone, it stands to reason that sedation dentistry is a good option for many people.

Whether or not it is the right option for your family depends on the factors involved, including the level of fear and anxiety present, how their overall health is, and what their doctor recommendation would be. Also, it's important to make sure that if you are considering it, you speak to the dentist and get all the details regarding what to do beforehand, what to expect during it, and what will happen once it is over. Only when you have all the information can you make an informed decision that will be the right one for you and your family.

Finding the right dentist is essential, especially if you are considering sedation dentistry. It's an area that plays an important role for millions of people, and one that the dentist needs to be experienced and knowledgeable about. Only you will know if choosing sedation dentistry is the right route, but at least now you know more about it and can use this information in helping to make your decision.

CHAPTER 11

When to Consider Cosmetic or Implant Dentistry

There are millions of people who are walking around with missing teeth. As we have discussed in prior chapters, there are many people who have dental problems and don't get them addressed. When that happens, they tend to lose the teeth, and often people will continue to leave them like that. They may be missing one tooth or they may be missing multiple ones, but millions of people are missing teeth.

We know that when you are missing teeth it can have devastating consequences. Those who are missing teeth tend to not be confident, because they know it doesn't look the best. They may end up hiding their mouth when they speak or laugh, and they may shy away from being in social groups. Teeth are something that people always look at in another person, and they help to give someone personality. One's teeth are their signature, if you will, or their unique fingerprint. Everyone has their own unique set of teeth and it helps to create who you are and what you look like.

When teeth are missing, there are going to be other problems even beyond the confidence issue. There can be health problems that arise as well. Teeth work together in what I like to think of as a team atmosphere. They all work together to give you the set of teeth you have. When there is one or more missing, there will be more of a strain or stress put on the others. The teeth next to where the open space is often shift to accommodate for the empty space. This can be devastating to the entire row of teeth, because it creates a dominoes-like shift in the mouth.

If you are someone who is missing teeth, or someone in your family is, what should you do? Is it best for you to continue ignoring it or just getting by, or is there a better route? Well, I'm glad you asked, because there is certainly a better route. The more you learn about the options available to help address a missing tooth, the better prepared you will be to get the situation taken care of. In this chapter, we will explore the options that are out there for you, including cosmetic and implant dentistry.

COSMETIC DENTISTRY

There are millions of people each year who opt for cosmetic dentistry. This is because cosmetic dentistry can be a great way to enhance your appearance, turbocharge our confidence, as well as compliment your overall health, and help to maintain your oral health. Cosmetic dentistry can help you improve tooth function, as well as help you love your smile.

There are numerous procedures that are included under the umbrella of cosmetic dentistry. Some of these procedures include bonding, implants, bridges, dentures, braces, periodontal plastic surgery, crowns, veneers, teeth whitening, and tooth-colored fillings. There are many options available, and each depends on what you may need and what your overall oral health goals may be. You may be a good candidate for some these procedures, but it's always good to discuss it with your trusted dentist. This is one more reminder why it is so important to have the best dentist for you. It's important that you have complete trust in your dentist and that you feel they will be making the best recommendations for you and putting your best interests ahead.

Let's look at a few of these popular common cosmetic dentistry options that are available today.

BONDING

Bonding is a popular option that involves a filling material that is attached to the original tooth. This is an ideal option for those who have a chipped or broken tooth, or someone who has a tooth that is improperly shaped. For those who have a tooth that is peg-shaped or smaller than it should be, this is a good option to consider. The filling material is bonded to the original tooth enamel and dentin, so that it looks and feels natural. It also functions like your regular tooth, so you will feel comfortable with using the tooth that has bonding. Tooth bonding is a procedure that offers a great way to help repair chipped teeth or address other issues.

DENTURES

There are several options when it comes to dentures, including partial dentures, full dentures, and overdentures. Some forms of dentures have been used for many years. Depending on how many teeth are missing or the types of gum conditions that someone may have, dentures may be a good option. Partial dentures are used when someone is missing groups of teeth, while full dentures are used to replace both teeth and gums. Overdentures are a newer option in the world of dentures. The process of using overdentures involves having implants put in that help to keep the denture in place. It's believed that overdentures may also help with better long-term success, because it may help eliminate bone loss where the implants are located.

PORCELAIN CROWNS

A solid choice for those who have a damaged tooth, porcelain crowns are made to fit over the damaged tooth, down to the gum. It provides a strong and resilient tooth covering that looks natural and functions like your regular tooth. Those who get large fillings may be a good option for getting porcelain crown inlays or onlays. The inlays are porcelain put over the grooves and cusp tip, while the onlays are often used to give a new look to an old filling. The porcelain color can be made to match the color of the tooth, helping to provide a natural look.

PORCELAIN FIXED BRIDGES

Porcelain options are a popular choice in cosmetic dentistry. They offer durability and they look great, making more people feel comfortable having them. A porcelain fixed bridge is an option that is available for someone who is missing one or more teeth. The porcelain fixed bridge is created to look just like the natural tooth that it is replacing, usually creating a flawless look to a problem area.

PORCELAIN VENEERS

Creating a natural smile is easier when you opt for procedures such as porcelain veneers. Sometimes veneers are called "instant orthodontics" because we can give you a perfect smile in just a few appointments, instead of years of braces. Again, porcelain provides strength and durability, while helping to create a natural look. Thin pieces of porcelain are used to replace your original tooth enamel. They adhere right to the tooth, giving your tooth a nice, natural look and natural function. To put them on, a tiny amount of enamel from the tooth is removed. They are a popular option for those who may have a discolored tooth or have issues with the shape of their tooth, as well as those who have overlaps or small gaps. With veneers, your own teeth stay intact for the most part, and they resist stains from such things as coffee, tea, and smoking cigarettes. The one drawback that you need to be aware of when considering porcelain veneers is that it is not considered reversible, because a tiny amount of enamel on the teeth was removed in order to put them on.

TOOTH-COLORED FILLINGS

Years ago, people got metal fillings. Today there are millions of people who have several metal fillings in their mouth. Often times they need to be replaced over time, and other times people want a better look. Rather than opening their mouth to laugh and showing their metal fillings, they are opting for tooth-colored fillings. Whether you are getting a filling for the first time, are replacing an old one that is worn out, or you want to enhance your look, tooth-colored fillings are an ideal choice. The composite resins and porcelains that are used today for fillings help to keep the metal out of the mouth and provide a more natural look and feel.

TEETH WHITENING

Nobody wants to have a smile that shows teeth stained from coffee, tea, or cigarette smoking, among other things. There are plenty of options available today for whitening your teeth, which will give you the confidence you want and need, and help create a more beautiful smile. While there are products available in the stores, they will never compare in quality to what your dentist can offer. Teeth whitening is an affordable cosmetic dentistry option for those who want to enhance their look. There are several types of dentist-provided teeth whitening options available today, including both in-office and at-home approaches. In-office teeth whitening will focus on using a stronger whitening agent, while still protecting the tooth. In just one visit, you can see a difference in the color of your teeth, often brightening several shades with just one application. Depending on how well you take care of your teeth, the whitening that you have done can last for a year or even several years before needing it done again to maintain your brighter smile. Your dentist can provide you with such things as custom fitted mouth trays for whitening your teeth, which will give you a more successful whitening. Most people believe that whiter teeth are more appealing, which makes teeth whitening one of the most common cosmetic dentistry options there is. It's usually an option that is affordable, easy to do, provides good results, and one that helps people love their smile and feel more confident showing it off.

BRACES

Braces can be both cosmetic and a medical necessity. You are going to have a perfect smile, and you will avoid problems that misaligned teeth can cause. No longer just for pre-teens, there are millions of adults even getting braces today. Not only are they a great way to help give you the beautiful smile that you want, but they will also help protect your overall oral health by addressing problems. While traditional metal braces are available, there are other more discreet options available today, including clear aligners that you can take out for an hour per day in order to eat and brush your teeth. The field has come a long way in terms of straightening teeth, and you may find that you want to get the braces that you should have had a couple of decades ago.

There are numerous options available today in cosmetic dentistry. If you have issues that you want addressed, you should explore your options. Speak with the dentist to see if they feel it is also a good fit for your situation, and explore all of the options that they offer at that office. As technology continuously changes, new procedures emerge. Even if there isn't an option that appeals to you today, there is a good chance that one may appeal to you in the near future. Like other areas in life, the dental industry is always changing, as we look for ways to improve people's lives through good oral health and a beautiful smile.

IMPLANT DENTISTRY

If you are like most people your age you don't give much thought to the health of your teeth or putting money into it to make improvements. You are probably content in life, just getting by with what you have, and assuming that this is just the way things are. Sure, you go for the minimum appointments and do what you need to in order to get by, but a great dentist will want you to get far more out of life than just getting by. You want to be able to have a better quality of life and keep your health good for as long as you can.

The scientific community already knows that poor dental health leads to poor overall health, which gives people a diminished quality of life. With something as simple as implant dentistry we help hold the key to what can combat that diminished quality of life. Implant dentistry can help you feel whole again, giving you the ability to enjoy more of the things that make you smile. Whether it's enjoying an ear of corn on the cob, or not having to put your teeth into a cup in the bathroom each night, implant dentistry can do wonders for you and your health.

The most common excuse that people give for not investing in implant dentistry is that they don't want to spend the money on it. For some reason, they don't feel their health and well-being is worth investing in. They are all saving up for a rainy day that never seems to come, or they are saving it to give to someone else after they pass on. Well, I'm here to say that you absolutely deserve to be happy and healthy right now. You deserve and owe it to yourself to invest in your own health and well-being. You are worth investing in.

Worth having its own category, implant dentistry has become increasingly popular in recent years. Implants can be the best thing dentistry has to offer for you, if they are right for you. It's important to know all you can about it if you will be considering it as an option for you or someone in your family. Implant dentistry helps people obtain a fuller, more natural-looking smile and it offers some benefits as well.

Implant dentistry started in Sweden, when a team led by Dr. P.I. Branemark learned that titanium can bond with bone. Implant dentistry involves using a small threaded screw that is made out of titanium. The screw is implanted into your gum where your missing tooth is, and a crown is put over the end of the implant, which looks like your natural tooth and fits in with your other teeth. If you have a missing tooth and you don't have anything there to continue to stabilize the bone, it will lead to more damage. The bone that holds your teeth in place is essentially dissolved away once you lose a tooth. This can create a shift in your teeth and lead to additional tooth loss and gum problems.

When that happens, it can lead to problems with everything from your bite and how you chew to your facial appearance. Once your teeth begin to shift, it can have a dramatic impact on how you look. It can even impact how you speak. Some people who experience this go on to become withdrawn, because they are so embarrassed by what has happened and how they look, and they also end up having health problems due to poor nutrition. The shift and loss of teeth can have a detrimental effect on what people eat, thus leading to a poor diet.

Today, the success rate is around 96 percent, making the implants a great choice for most people. There are a few factors that need to be considered before opting for dental implants. It is believed that doctors who do more implants each year have a higher success rate, which stands to reason. Therefore, it's important to choose a dentist who is well experienced in doing implants. You want one who does over fifty implants per year, so that you will have a higher success rate from their being experienced.

Another factor that will be considered is the person's bone quality. The dentist will need to implant the screw into the bone, so there needs to be a minimal amount there in order to perform the procedure. This doesn't mean that if you already have bone loss there that it's too late for implants. Through sophisticated procedures, well-experienced dentists can perform bone grafting in order to help you have the bone needed for the procedure. Typically, the bone would come from your own lower jaw, or it can even be taken from other sources, such as bovine bone or cadavers.

If you are considering having implants done, the dentist is going to need to know your medical history. A clinical exam and thorough medical history will be taken, so that they can be sure that you don't have any conditions that would create complications for the implants or for the medical conditions you have. Some of the medical problems that could be of concern include liver disease, diabetes, and bleeding disorders. If you have any of these conditions and are still interested in implant dentistry, speak with your trusted dentist. That's the only way to find out if it's a good fit for you or if there are better options with the conditions that you have.

With implants, there is a healing phase that can take up to six months. During that time, you will never be without your teeth, so you will still be comfortable and your mouth will be fully functioning. Once your implants are finished and healed, it's important to continue to take good care of them, just as you would your own natural teeth. Just like your natural teeth, they can develop bone loss, as well as gingivitis. You will need to brush and floss them daily, just as your natural teeth, as well as go for regular cleanings and exams. The implant offers a long-term solution that lasts for many years, and it will help you to maintain your jawbone, which is a huge benefit in protecting your overall oral and general health

There are some dentists who offer implant dentistry. If they do, it's a service that requires additional training in order to provide it. Many people go to a specialist for implants, such as a periodontist, or oral and maxillofacial surgeons. In choosing where to have yours done, be sure that the office is well experienced and is qualified to be offering the service. You can expect to pay around $3,000, or more, per tooth, which doesn't include additional fees if you need bone grafting or the crown that will go on the titanium screw. Although you want to be aware of the average cost, the cost shouldn't be the most important factor. You must have a credentialed doctor perform the work, so make that your highest priority when deciding who will do it. You want quality work by a well-experienced dentist, not the cheapest price you can find. There is a lot at stake, and it needs to be done right in order for you to have long-term success.

MAKING THE DECISION

When it comes to whether or not cosmetic dentistry is the right fit for you and your family, you have a few things to consider. For starters, what your overall goals are in getting it. Consider whether or not it's going to add a better quality of life, help protect your overall health, or if it will be beneficial in other ways.

Your teeth are such an important part of your life, your character, and in your overall health, that considering cosmetic or implant dentistry makes good sense. If you are someone who is missing teeth, has worn-out crowns, has a chipped tooth, wants to replace metal crowns, or would like to have teeth that just look better, there is an option for you. Today's cosmetic dentistry field is high-tech, advanced, and provides many options that will give you a beautiful smile that looks and feels natural. It will help you get the most out of your teeth for the long haul, and help to protect your overall health and confidence level.

Increasingly there are insurance companies that are paying for cosmetic dentistry and implant options. They realize that there are many benefits to people getting the procedures done. If you are concerned about the costs associated with cosmetic dentistry or getting implants, be sure to check with your insurance provider first to see what is covered and what options they offer, and speak with the dentist to see what options they can recommend.

Remember, getting dental work done may be seen as expensive, but it pales in comparison to the expense of not getting the work done. Finding the right dentist for you so that you get the best treatment is essential. Make it a priority and your dental needs will be met in a way that keeps you smiling for many years to come.

CHAPTER 12

Choose a Highly Successful Dentist

By this point, you know that choosing the right dentist for you and your family is crucial. There is a lot at stake, and you don't want to get it wrong. Far too often, people don't pay much attention to which dentist they choose, only to be disappointed once they have an appointment or two. Treat choosing a dentist as something highly important, because believe me, it is. It's more important than most people tend to realize, and it can have far-reaching consequences if you don't get it right.

Not having the right dentist at your side can lead to host of problems, many of which we have covered in this book. If you are with the wrong dentist, it can make you and your family want to back away from getting the treatment that they need. Appointments may be skipped, dreaded, or you may have anxiety about each one, making it difficult for to keep up with the routine. When it comes to your kids, you are creating a foundation for the relationship they will likely forever have with the dental world. The choices you make today could set them up to either fear and avoid going to the dentist later in life, or it could help them become more comfortable and feel that it's an important part of their overall health.

We already know there are devastating consequences to having poor oral health. When people have poor oral health, it affects their mental health, as well as their physical health. Children who have a poor oral health image will usually suffer from an increase in being bullied and become more withdrawn. It can make them not want to participate in social interactions and even refrain from participating in school as they should.

Adults who have poor oral health can go on to have poor general health. There will also be social problems because of the dental image issues, including that they are more embarrassed, less confident, and may even get passed over for jobs and promotions. Those who don't care for their teeth or smile will usually try to hide it when they laugh or talk, making it difficult for them to participate in social interactions as they would like to. It can also have devastating effects on being able to find dates and romantic partners. There are many great reasons for making your oral health a huge priority in your life, and not one good reason not to.

Just about every parent wants to help give their child the best start in life that they can. We want to protect them, help them learn to do the right thing, take good care of their health, and go on to become productive and successful adults. One thing we can do in helping us achieve those goals is to ensure that their dental needs are successfully met, so that they don't ever experience the life-changing problems that can arise from them not liking their teeth or smile.

As parents, we owe it to our children to help protect their teeth by ensuring they have the best dentist in their court. When they have a great dentist at their side, they will feel more comfortable knowing that the recommendations, treatments, and steps taken are in the best interest of the child. Children aside, you also deserve to have a great dentist. While I don't know what you have personally been through in your life when it comes to your dental experience, I can say without a doubt that I have come in contact with thousands of patients in my life. I have seen and heard it all, and I have also fixed it all, often times fixing what wasn't done right elsewhere.

When you find the right dentist, you will know it. You will have no doubt about it. You will feel it and you will no longer question whether you should continue on or look for another. Once you have the right dentist you come to have a sense of trust, and being in anyone else's chair simply won't do. Any other dentist you ever meet will be measured up against that one that you know is different, stands out, and is highly successful. Your mission is to find a dentist who is highly successful. And if you choose to accept that mission, you will be successful at it.

DEFINING HIGHLY SUCCESSFUL

To some extent, you could say that every dentist is successful. After all, they did go through dental school and they have succeeded in becoming a dentist in the first place. But that's about where it ends. Everything beyond that is going to be what separates those who simply made it as a dentist and those who have gone on to become highly successful dentists. As you can imagine, there are going to be a lot fewer highly successful dentists out there than there are simply dentists.

Many people who finish dental school either get a job in someone else's office, or they hang out their own shingle to open their practice. This puts them in business and they can start seeing patients. But that doesn't mean that they are a great dentist, have the experience you want or need, or even care about being highly successful.

For starters, let me tell you what a good dentist is like. A good dentist will meet your needs when you go, and give you exactly what you expected. That good dentist will do exactly what you assumed would be done, and treat you exactly how you thought you would or should be treated. And then there won't be much more beyond that. They don't feel they need to do anything else beyond that. After all, they are a good dentist, and the patients seem to be satisfied and continue to come back.

Now let me tell you what it's like when you see a highly successful dentist. They won't stop at just meeting your needs. They know that meeting your needs and giving you what you expect should be the minimum that you get when you go to the dentist. When you go the office of a highly successful dentist, you will find that the bare minimum, or just meeting your expectations, will never do. They will always strive for more and will always go above and beyond. At their office, they want to know your name, the things you care about, they want to create a relationship with you, and they want you walking out feeling like you were a star visiting their office that day. They treat everyone like gold, because they realize how important every patient is. They want you to feel special and they will always go out of their way to treat you like they would treat their own family. How's that for exceptional dental care?

Why would ever want to go do a dentist's office that just meets your expectations? Of course they should do that. They don't have to do much in order to meet your expectations, so they are not putting forth much effort. You deserve going to a dentist's office where they will always thumb their nose at the idea of just meeting expectations. You want the red carpet treatment, you want to feel like you belong there, and you want to feel understood and listened to. You want all of your questions answered about treatments and procedures, and you don't want the dentist keeping one eye on the clock as those questions are being answered.

Believe it or not, there are highly successful dentists out there, and one of them is waiting for you to become their patient. You didn't realize they exist, but now that you do, it should become a priority to find one for you and your family. You will love the difference that each appointment makes in how you feel when you have a highly successful dentist who genuinely cares about the patients, their best needs, rises above just meeting expectations, and treats patients like they would treat their own family. When you find that person, you have found the right dentist. Hold on tight, and make the best of every appointment. You and your family will enjoy the ride, rather than dreading every dentist appointment as you likely do now.

Pay attention from the start to see how well you are treated not only from the dentist, but everyone in their office. The entire team should be on board with being committed to providing exceptional care to each and every patient. Even when you make the first phone call to inquire about setting up an appointment or to ask questions regarding their services, you should feel it that they are a great place. If, on the other hand, you place that call and they seem aloof, as if they don't care if you become a patient, they are not eager to get you into their office, and the kindness doesn't come through, see it as a red flag. We want better than just having expectations met or being just okay. Anyone can be just okay, but someone who meets that standard will never be the best possible dentist for you and your family. You and your family deserve much better than just okay. In fact, the health of your mouth and overall health are depending on it being better than just okay.

The team in a highly successful dentist's office will also be top notch. The dentist will know the value of an exceptional team and will invest in them. They will know what the goals are, what is expected of them in terms of customer service, and they will have had the proper training in order to provide exemplary service. Only highly successful dentists realize this, and will make the effort to create a stellar team and office atmosphere.

ADDITIONAL EXCEPTIONAL QUALITIES

The commitment to excellent patient care and going above and beyond for everyone in the chair are not the only qualities that make for a highly successful dentist. That's certainly a big piece of the puzzle of what makes someone highly successful, but there are additional exceptional qualities you can look for. Some of the common personality traits of a highly successful dentist include:

- **Being easy to talk to and being a good listener**. A dentist needs to help put people at ease and calm fears and anxiety. They can easily do this through the things they say to help the patient. They can also do this by thoroughly answering questions and explaining in detail what the patient can expect. They should have no problems with working closely with others. As you realize, a dentist has to work in close contact with their patients. If someone is uncomfortable with that, it will make it difficult for them to be a great dentist. They will continuously be worried about pulling back and having more space away from the person.

- **A sense of trustworthiness**. Patients need to learn to trust their dentist in order to have a great relationship. The best way that this is done is through honest and open communication where the dentist takes the patient's needs and concerns into account and helps them work through each one. It may take patience to work with each patient, but the dentist who has it and demonstrates it will help build trust.

- **Someone who is a passionate about what they do**. They didn't go into the profession to get rich, because unless their heart and soul are in it, they likely never will. Only those dentists who are truly passionate about what they do and about helping people achieve their dental goals will become highly successful. A dentist who is excited about the field will continue to keep up on new trends, technology, and will want to continue furthering their skills and knowledge, so that it can be put to good use helping their patients.

- **A highly successful dentist must be a great communicator and effective leader**. Not just with each patient, but with everyone they come in contact with. A dental office can only be highly successful if the dentist has a great team working in the office who can effectively carry out the mission. Often times, it is the team of professionals at the dentist's office that you will be spending some time with, and each one needs to help reassure you that they value you as a patient. They also need to be great at communication, so they can help you with appointments, concerns, billing, etc. It takes a team of great people to help create a highly successful dentist. The dentist can't do it all on their own.

- **Someone who is detailed-oriented and organized**. Dental procedures often require a lot of steps and deal with small items. It's imperative that the dentist be detailed oriented in order to get it right.

- **A highly successful dentist must have a sense of caring about their patients**. They cannot be so absorbed in the work that they forget to ask the patient how they are doing or ask if they need a break. Showing that they care about the patient speaks volumes about their sense of compassion and understanding and will go a long way toward helping patients to feel comfortable.

- **It also helps for a dentist to have some artistic skills**. After all, they are helping to create a beautiful smile, so being able to master certain techniques to help them do that is a highly desirable attribute.

Chances are, you never thought much about what qualities may be needed to be a highly successful dentist. But each of these listed above play an important role in helping to give you an exceptional dental experience. Without them, you would notice and you would not be happy or completely satisfied as a patient. With them, you will feel like you have finally found the best possible dentist for you and you will not believe what an awesome difference it will make in your life and in your oral health.

MORE HIGHLY SUCCESSFUL QUALITIES

There are some additional things you can look for that will help set the highly successful dentists apart. Some of these things include teaching other dentists at conferences, college courses, or through continuing education. Not only do highly successful dentists continue to keep learning all the latest in the field, but they share with others.

Highly successful dentists will also be published. They will have most likely have articles and books that they have published, offering information to the masses. They will have been quoted in articles put out by others, demonstrating their commitment to the community and the faith the journalists have in their skills and abilities.

Some of the other things that highly successful dentists do are giving back to their community, and being an active part of it. They host events so that they can help the community come together and celebrate, have fun, and be a part of something. They also help those less fortunate in a variety of ways. Whether helping to support something that is going on at a local school, or making mission trips to provide free dental care to those in third world countries.

In addition to being highly skilled and educated, there are many interpersonal and community-related skills and experiences that come together to make for a highly successful dentist.

The dentists who stand out, rise above, and reach the highest levels of success are well-rounded individuals who are surrounded by an amazing team. They are well respected by their peers, have patients who are fiercely loyal, and will always go above and beyond for every one of their patients.

The best and most successful dentists out there cover all bases. They know how to be an effective leader to their team, how to prioritize their business, and are committed to integrity in their business. They plan for success, achieve goals, and continue to move the line of what they will accomplish next. They stay hungry for wanting to do more in their field and help as many patients as possible.

Being highly successful is a combination of hard work, dedication to the field, a commitment to excellence, learning from setbacks, and perseverance. There isn't one description that can be given for what a highly successful dentist is, because it's a combination of things. Skills, education, teaching others, and going above and beyond are all necessary, but they need to be combined with the best personality characteristics in order for the dentist to make a connection with the people. Someone can be very successful on paper, for example, and yet lack in the social skills department, which makes their patients not feel comfortable or informed.

It's important to choose a highly successful dentist. It's part of choosing the best possible dentist for you and your family. Now you have a better sense of what to look for in terms of success. Look beyond the signs and ads and see what the dentist has done and how the person treats those around them and how they fit in with the community.

CHAPTER 13

What Can I Expect at the Initial Consultation and Exam?

The moment you step into the dentist's office, you know just how important it was that you took the time to find the right one for you and your family. The energy in the office atmosphere will usually tell you a lot. It can either put you at ease or scare the daylights out of you. The last thing you want is to step into that office only to find yourself nervously waiting for your name to be called. Worse yet, you don't want to be choked up and start getting those little beads of perspiration once you do get called and make your way back to the exam room.

Taking the time to find the best possible dentist is going to help eliminate the fears and put you at ease. You will no longer cringe at the thought of having an appointment. Nor will you sit there biting your nails as you wait for your name to be called. No, once you have found the right dentist you will relax, unwind, and find ways to enjoy spending those few minutes in the waiting area. Whether flipping through a magazine or reading a few pages in the book you are currently reading, you will have no more worries at the thought of your appointments.

Your initial consultation and exam is going to create the foundation for the relationship you have with that dentist office. First impressions are a big, big deal.

Many people wonder what to expect when they go for their initial consultation and exam. Fair enough. The more you know what to expect, the less anxiety you will feel as the clock moves closer to your appointment time. Being prepared for what is going to take place helps put people at ease. While it may be helpful for you, it's also a good idea to speak with children about what to expect, to help eliminate their fears. We'll get to that a little later in this chapter, so you have an idea of what to say to get them off to a great start with the dentist.

YOUR FIRST APPOINTMENT

Once you have done the necessary research and evaluation in order to find what you believe is going to be the best dentist for you and your family, it's time to make the first appointment. While the process may vary somewhat at each dental office, there are some standard things that should take place at your first consultation and exam.

Here's a breakdown of those things so you have an idea of what to expect should take place.

1. **Greeting**. The first thing that should happen when you arrive is that you should be properly greeted. Everyone who works in the dentist's office should be well trained and know how to treat every patient. Since they are expecting you, they should have things prepared and be ready for you when you arrive. You will have some paperwork to complete so that they have your contact information and some medical history. Many times they will offer those papers to you over the phone when you make the appointment. If they email them to you or tell you where to find them on their website to download and print them off, you can show up for the appointment with them already filled out. Many people find this a more convenient way to get the paperwork done, rather than trying to get it done on the spot when they show up for the appointment. The paperwork they ask you to fill out is typically required by law and is a standard procedure across practices.

2. **Tour**. Its important to get a tour of the office, so you can be familiar with everything it has to offer, including technology, check out, and even the patient bathroom.

3. **X-rays**. Your initial exam is going to usually include X-rays, unless there are issues that would prevent them, such as your age or diseases. Those who are pregnant are also usually excluded from getting X-rays, unless there is an emergency situation making it necessary to have them. By getting X-rays of the mouth and jawbones, the dentist can often find issues that cannot be detected with

the naked eye. X-rays are helpful for helping to diagnose such conditions as cysts, tumors, impacted teeth, jawbone damage, and decay taking place in between teeth. During the first appointment, the dentist will often take a series of X-rays, including a panoramic one, which will give the dentist a good view of both the upper and lower jaw on one film. This type of X-ray is helpful because it shows your bite and how your teeth fit together. The dentist will usually show you the X-rays and go over them with you, pointing out any issues that are of concern.

4. **Photography**. A great way to see exactly what is happening in your mouth, and to see exactly what the dentist is seeing, is through digital photography. During the exam, you will sit knee to knee with the dentist, to see exactly what he is seeing when he looks in your mouth.

5. **Examination**. Your dentist will conduct a full examination of your mouth. They will be looking at the teeth and gums, and also any specific areas of concern that have been identified by the X-rays or that you have mentioned. The dentist may identify problems or areas of concern even though you may not be aware of them yet. The goal of every dentist is to find the problems early on, so they can be addressed and they can help keep them from becoming bigger problems later on. The sooner you treat issues, the better off you will be. Dental problems don't tend to go away, they usually start small and continue to worsen over time. The worse they get, the bigger procedure it usually is to address them, and they can go on to negatively impact other teeth, gums, or your jawbone.

6.   **Cleaning**. Your initial dentist visit will usually also include a thorough cleaning with the hygienist or with the dentist. They will use special instruments to remove any build-up of plaque on or in between the teeth, scrape below the gumline, and they will usually floss and polish your teeth. During this cleaning they will usually evaluate the health of your gums. This is usually a painless process. The test they use to check the health of your gums is called a periodontal chart. They determine the health of your gums, which correlates with the numbers on the periodontal chart by measuring in millimeters (mm) the depth of the cuff of gum tissue that surrounds each tooth. As they check this, you will usually hear the person doing the evaluation saying numbers as another person records each one. The lower the number for each tooth, the better the health of that gum area is. For example, if a tooth has a 0-3 mm space without bleeding, then there are no issues and it's a healthy gum. A 3-5 mm with bleeding, on the other hand, is considered early to moderate gum disease, or the beginning of periodontitis. Those teeth with a 7 mm and above rating are considered to have advanced periodontal disease and aggressive treatment will be needed. It's important to keep in mind that healthy gums do not bleed, so if yours are bleeding during the cleaning, exam, or even when you are brushing and flossing at home, there is an issue that needs to be treated. During the initial appointment, your dentist should evaluate for this and if there is a problem will discuss treatment options with you.

At some dentist's offices, the office manager or the treatment coordinator (your new patient assistant) will sit down with you to go over your needs. This usually comes after having your exam and cleaning. This is the time that they will discuss such issues as insurance and pricing with you. Be sure to ask questions you may have, including those about payment options. The office manager will be able to discuss the variety of options that are available for payment for the treatment that you may need. They can also answer insurance-related questions.

Once your dentist has been able to review the X-rays and to examine your mouth, they will know if there are issues of concern. If there are problems identified, such as issues with the gums, cavities, or other areas of concern, your dentist will likely recommend treatment options to you. They should be thorough in providing you with the information you need regarding what the treatment involves, how long it takes, and what you can expect from the outcome. Be sure to ask any questions you may have. A great dentist will answer all of your questions and want you to be comfortable knowing exactly what is going on and what to expect.

If you have issues that need to be addressed, and especially if you have multiple ones, your dentist will create a treatment plan for you. This will give you an idea of all of the things you need done, as well as the costs associated with them. There may be pressing issues that need to be handled right away, because they are bothering you, and there may be ones that you may be able to plan out down the line. Having a treatment plan will help get you on the right course to having the work done that you need in order to have a healthy mouth. You should be given a copy of your treatment plan to take home with you. This helps keep you informed, so that you know exactly what you need done and the costs associated with each treatment. If you are not given a treatment plan to take home, be sure to ask for a copy.

If you need treatment for a condition, they will usually make a follow-up appointment for that. If they have the time and it's a quick procedure, it may be something they can do right then. At this point you will make your appointment for the treatment, or if there were no issues you will make your next routine appointment. For those who don't have problems or concerns, you will typically have an appointment every four to six months. Once per year, you will have the X-rays and meet with the dentist for an exam, while on the other appointments you may only meet with the hygienist for a cleaning.

It's always better to address dental issues right away. Waiting to have them looked at or treated usually leads to them getting worse.

At your six-month checkup, you may only see the hygienist for a cleaning if you didn't have any areas of concern during the last appointment. However, your hygienist should ask you if you have had any problems, pain, or concerns. If you have, share them with the hygienist, who will pass that info on to the dentist. If there have been concerns, the dentist should come in and take a look and further evaluate the situation. You also should not wait until your next six-month appointment if you have problems in between appointments. If there are problems that arise, whether it is a hurting tooth, bleeding gums, or something else, give the dentist a call and have it evaluated right away.

Many people have questions that they would love to ask their dentist or hygienist, or even the front office staff, yet they shy away from it. Don't take those questions home with you. Always ask the questions you have on your mind. I can tell you that in my office we have never minded answering questions. In fact, we want to. We want every one of our patients to feel comfortable asking questions, we want them to feel well informed, and we never want them to walk out of our office wishing they could have asked us something. Speak up, let us know, ask us, and find out. That's what we are there for, and we can't give you the info you need if you don't take the time to tell us what is on your mind or what you may be concerned with.

TALKING WITH CHILDREN

As discussed earlier on, it is important to get it right with children from the start. By that, I mean it is critical that a healthy relationship with the dentist be formed right from the start. Their first experiences are going to lay the foundation for how they feel about going to the dentist for years, maybe even into adulthood. This is why it's important to help lay a healthy foundation regarding the dentist at home, before you even step foot into their office for an appointment.

Believe it or not, parents often scare children about going to the dentist, and they instill in them an unnecessary fear. Most of the time they don't even realize they are doing this, but children are very perceptive. They pick up on your attitudes and fears about the dentist and will internalize them, making them their own. Plus, parents may say things like, "Brush your teeth or they will fall out," or, "The dentist is going to be drilling your teeth." These can be scary thoughts to children, making them afraid of the dentist.

According to the American Academy of Pediatric Dentistry, your child should start seeing a dentist by the time their first tooth appears, or by their first birthday. Some people raise their eyebrows at this being so early, but this is the best way to get a head start on preventing dental problems. Caught early on, dentists can help you avoid problems becoming worse and help prevent serious issues.

Healthy dental care for children begins with the appearance of their first tooth.

Parents can help children get comfortable with going to the dentist starting with the things they say. For starters, pay attention to how you speak about going to the dentist yourself. Avoid speaking about any pain from the treatment in front of your children (if there is any pain or discomfort). Focus on the positives and use terms that let your child know that the dentist helped you, is there to help keep your teeth healthy, and try to keep things simple. They won't understand complex details about treatments, so it's best to keep things simple.

Along the lines of watching what you say about going to the dentist in front of your children, it's important to keep your own childhood dental stories in check if they weren't happy ones. The dental field has come a long way over the years, and today there are treatment options that aim to help keep kids comfortable. There's no need to share those stories, which may instill fear in them about going to the dentist.

The main words you want to avoid when speaking with children about going to the dentist are shot, pain, and hurt. If they hear those words, they will not want to go to the dentist. Parents can help their child become comfortable with the idea of going to the dentist by having a pretend trial run, where the parent pretends to be the dentist. They can also get a book or two that has a story about going to the dentist. It's good to talk to them about going and the importance of taking care of their teeth, but it needs to be done in simple terms and on a positive note.

If you have children, you will want to make sure you are choosing a dentist's office that is kid-friendly. Not all of them are, so even if you feel you have found a great dentist it may not be a good fit for kids. Some dentists don't begin seeing children until they are a certain age, such as five or even ten. Those with children will find that they are better off going to a pediatric dentist's office. A pediatric dentist is someone who has had 2-3 years of additional specialty training beyond dental school, where they have focused on treating children.

When you do take your child for their appointment, be sure to focus on the positives and try to curb any fears they may have. The staff at the office should know to focus on making it a positive experience for the child. With smaller children, you may still find some squirming. That's to be expected, and the dentist office staff may know some tricks of the trade to get them focused and calmed down. Again, be sure to ask questions so that you get the information you need in being able to give your child the best treatment plan and help put them on the path to good oral hygiene.

FIRST APPOINTMENTS MATTER

Your first appointment at a new dentist's office is a big deal. You know it and so does the dentist. You may have done all your evaluating and researching to find the best possible dentist, but it's that first appointment that tells you if your assessment was correct. That one appointment should help put you at ease and let you know that you made the right choice. If it doesn't, then there is a good chance you didn't do a thorough job of evaluating and choosing an office.

Your first dental appointment is a great time to start a new chapter in your dental life. This is a time for you to create a new relationship with the dentist, regardless of what your past experiences have been like. Go into it with a positive energy, knowing that you have done the research necessary to find a great one. Trust the work you did and the pick you made. With the right dentist, you will find that you actually don't mind going in for your appointments and that your teeth look better than ever.

Your dentist is your partner in helping to keep your teeth looking great and your oral health in good condition. With the right dentist, you will feel that right from the start. They are on your side, have your best interests in mind, and are ready to serve you and meet your needs.

CHAPTER 14

Why I am Your Dentist

Being passionate about the dental field, I take pride in being able to help people achieve great oral health and to have an amazing smile. When my patients are happy and have something to smile about in regard to their teeth, then I feel the same way. My success is tied to how they feel about the service and care that they are receiving from my office, so we go way above and beyond to provide the best possible care around.

Think back to all of the major things I have recommended to you in this book that your perfect dentist should have. Those things are all qualities that you will find in my office. Throughout the pages of this book, I have given you the tools, tips, and insider information you need so that you know what to look for when finding your best dentist. The information I have laid out in this book not only helped give you the confidence to evaluate and find the best possible dentist for you and your family, but it also put a spotlight on the reason it's so important for you to do so in the first place.

Finding the right dentist is not a matter to be taken lightly.

I've explained why your smile is so important, and what happens when you don't have a great smile or you have poor oral hygiene. I've also shared why a great smile is more than just a cosmetic issue, and why just any dentist will not do. It's imperative that you have the right dentist so that you will gain the most benefits. Your dental health is too important to gamble with.

In the pages of this book, I have advised that you choose a dentist who:

- Goes above and beyond for their patients and is grateful for every one of them.

- Has a well-trained team that knows exactly how to treat patients and why it's so important to make them a priority.

- Is highly successful and is a part of their community.

- Will take the time to answer all of your questions completely, explain treatments thoroughly, and be a good listener.

- Readily offers information about payment options, so that you can find a comfortable way to pay for the treatment that you and your family are in need of.

- Has a great reputation and is well-established in the field.

- Spends time both continuing to learn about advancements in the field and teaching them to other doctors and dental health professionals.

- Gives some of their time or resources to charity to help make the world a better place.

All of these things describe my practice and me. Not only am I an award-winning dental professional, but I also have an amazing team that has been well trained, and they understand the mission of carrying out my passion for providing excellence in dental care. At my offices, we always aim to go above and beyond, because just meeting expectations of our patients is not acceptable. We want to know every patient by name, who their favorite sports team is, and what they are passionate about. In other words, we care about the person and not just their mouth.

When you have your list of all the things you are looking for in the best dentist, you can easily check them off when you consider my practice and me. We know exactly what it takes to have a great practice and we go out of our way to make it happen. We stop at nothing short of striving to be the best in order to exceed expectations. Most of our new patients come by word-of-mouth, from others who speak so highly of our office. But I wouldn't want you to merely take someone else's word for it. As laid out in this book, I would want you to take the time to fully research and evaluate my office. I'm completely comfortable with you doing that, because I know without a doubt that we will come out ahead and pass every test with flying colors.

I know firsthand how life-changing great dental care can be. I've not only lived it myself, but I have seen the transformation that I've helped thousands of patients make. Having the right dentist can be a truly life-changing event. I've seen many people experience a surge in confidence following treatment. I've also seen people find the love of their life after the surge in confidence from having great teeth, as well as seen people get wonderful jobs.

Great things happen when you no longer feel you need to hide your smile or keep your mouth closed. When people feel great about their teeth, they will tend to smile more, be more outgoing, and the benefits and rewards of living like that just roll right in. Not only have I personally seen the vast life-changing differences that great treatment can give people, but I've heard the feedback, too. People often write or tell me about how their life changed following treatment in my office. Their great feedback puts a smile on my face and warms my heart, because it's exactly why we do what we do in our office.

The thorough initial exam that I explained in the prior chapter is what you can expect in my office. We are grateful for every new patient we get and we want to ensure that they are with us for a long time. We give them a thorough exam so that we can find any areas of concern and create a successful treatment plan for each and every patient. When it comes to being up front with the information and answering questions, we are dedicated to making sure you are comfortable and know exactly what your options are and what to expect. There are no surprises when it comes to the treatment that we are providing.

WHY CHOOSE US?

We literally wrote the book on what you should look for in an excellent dentist. You are holding it in your hand. Knowing what it takes to be the best and what you should want out of a dentist, we are committed to providing you with exactly that. Our office is comprised of a team of top-notch dental professionals who believe in what they do and are passionate about doing it well. From the first phone call to set up an appointment, you will be treated with the upmost respect. We try to meet your schedule and needs and always listen to the concerns you may have, so that everything can be addressed to your satisfaction.

We are your dentists, because we know exactly what you need in a great dentist and promise to provide it. Without our loyal list of patients, we don't have a practice. We have many happy patients and that is certainly not by accident or chance. We have earned every one of them through our commitment to them and the field. Our patients trust us to provide them with honest assessments, outstanding patient services, and excellent treatments. And that's what we aim to deliver to each and every patient who walks through our doors.

Whether you just need routine cleanings and exams or you would like to explore cosmetic dentistry options, we are able to handle all of your needs. Our team has done thousands of cosmetic dentistry procedures, including porcelain veneers, tooth whitening, tooth-colored fillings, porcelain fixed bridges, porcelain crowns, bonding, and braces. We are experts in the field, keep up on the latest technologies that will help improve treatments, and provide them with an unmatched professionalism.

If you are considering sedation dentistry, we are also happy to discuss those options with you. We always maintain keeping your best interest in mind and will discuss the variety options available to you and which ones we believe you are best suited for. We also have plenty of experience when it comes to tackling that ugly matter of money. We know that not everyone has a bank account big enough to write a check for all of the treatment that they may need. Our staff is ready with the payment option information that you need, to help make it easier for you to address your oral health and have the smile you dream of. Whether it is evaluating your current insurance, finding other plans that suit your needs, or providing payment option arrangements to consider, we are ready to help you every step of the way.

A crucial thing to remember about why I am your dentist is that I guarantee you will be happy. At our office, we always stand behind our work. If you are not happy with the treatment you have received, then we are not happy either, and we want everyone to be happy. While others may shy away from guaranteeing their work, we never do. We will always work tirelessly to ensure that are happy with the outcome of the treatments you receive. We wouldn't feel good about what we do if you walked out the door unhappy or dissatisfied with the outcome. Only when you are completely happy are we also happy. We will always stand behind our work.

We not only want you as a patient, but we care about you as a person. We want to make sure your oral health needs are met and that you love your smile. We want you to be comfortable and confident. Our mission is to be accessible to your needs. A great smile is more than just a cosmetic issue, as you have learned throughout the pages of this book. Your smile, whether good or not so good, impacts many areas of your life. We know that, so we make every effort to help you be the best version of yourself.

We know the science behind a smile, and we know the bullying and poor grades that come from not loving the one you have. Not having a nice smile can impact both children and adults, and it's an issue we are passionate about. We want to help everyone have a great smile so they can live a better quality of life and be confident enough to chase their dreams.

NOT JUST ANY DENTIST

In an earlier chapter, I urged you to not settle for just any old dentist. Resist the urge to make it easy by choosing the one who is closest to your house, who your friend goes to, or whose name showed up first in doing an online search. That is not enough criteria for you to choose a dentist. That's essentially throwing a dart at the wall and wherever it lands, that is who will be your dentist. You can do better than that, and you owe it to yourself to do better.

I know exactly what it takes to be an excellent dentist. My skills, experience, and passion for the field take me out of the equation of being just any old dentist. I continue to learn new technologies in the field, teach it to others through classes and seminars, and practice what I preach. I have thousands of patients who I have helped over the years. All of this has helped me become an award-winning dental professional. We start with a great first impression and it never diminishes from there. We believe in giving you patients the same great care that we would give to our own family members. After all, we see our team and patients as one big family.

Finally, I'd like to remind you how important personality is when choosing a dentist. Having a dentist you trust, can speak with, and feel comfortable with is huge. Given the opportunity, I am confident you will feel right at home in my office. I invite you to stop by my office and take a tour, meet the team, and see if you think we will be a great fit to be your next dentist.

If you find for some reason that we are not, maybe due to where you live, then I hope the information in this book will be helpful in finding the right dentist for you and your family. Whether my patient or not, I want you to have a dentist you love and teeth you feel confident and healthy with. I've laid out all of the information in this book that you need to find an awesome dentist who will be perfect for you and your family. Taking the time to do the research and evaluate will be time well spent.

My hope is that you finish this book feeling more confident about the importance of having a great dentist, what goes into finding one, and the steps you need to take in order make it happen. If you now feel more confident in being able to find a great dentist, then this book has served its intended purpose. I believe it would be a wonderful thing if everyone found the right dentist for them, and I'm happy to give people the blueprint to help make that happen.

I'm passionate about a great smile and helping others to have one. I have come to absolute conviction on this point: A person is either going through life smiling with confidence or hiding their smile with humiliation. We all make the decision, which we need to choose wisely. There's an old Chinese proverb that says "Use your smile to change the world; don't let the world change your smile." Your smile truly can be that powerful, and when you have the right dentist you can absolutely use your smile to change the world. We can help you have that powerful smile that you want and need.